YOU ARE WHAT YOU EAT...AND SMOKE.

Do you know that you would have to gain 75 to 90 pounds to come close to the kind of damage that smoking does to your body?

Do you know that smoking changes your body chemistry?

Do you know that food tastes better once you've quit smoking?

FACT: Foods rich in vitamin C are the ex-smoker's best friend.

FACT: Taking a brisk walk is a great substitute for smoking—and it burns calories too!

Know the facts—and learn   616:865

How to Quit Smoking Without Gaining Weight

A proven plan for fighting nicotine addiction

The American Lung Association® is the oldest voluntary health organization in the United States. Founded in 1904, the American Lung Association fights lung disease in all its forms, including asthma, tobacco control, and environmental health. Visit the American Lung Association website at www.lungusa.org.

Bess H. Marcus, Ph.D., has helped hundreds of women quit smoking and thousands of men and women to become regular exercisers. She is Director of Physical Activity Research at the Brown University Center for Behavioral and Preventive Medicine at The Miriam Hospital.

Jeffrey S Hampl, Ph.D., R.D., is Associate Professor of Nutrition at Arizona State University and a spokesperson for the American Dietetic Association.

Edwin B. Fisher, Ph.D., an ex-smoker himself, is the author of the best-selling *7 Steps to a Smoke-Free Life*. Dr. Fisher is Professor of Psychology, Medicine and Pediatrics at Washington University.

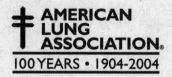

AMERICAN LUNG ASSOCIATION®

100 YEARS • 1904-2004

How to Quit Smoking Without Gaining Weight

Bess H. Marcus, Ph.D.,
Jeffrey S Hampl, Ph.D., R.D., and
Edwin B. Fisher, Ph.D.

POCKET BOOKS

NEW YORK LONDON TORONTO SYDNEY

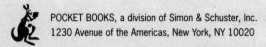

DEDICATIONS

Bess Marcus
To my husband, Dan, and my children, Brittany and Josh, for your love, laughter, and support.

Jeffrey Hampl
To my parents, Bill and Peg Hampl, for setting a good example.

Ed Fisher
For my mother, Eleanor Fisher, who shows how to live with health, energy, and optimism.

ACKNOWLEDGMENTS

The authors would like to thank Dr. Norman H. Edelman, Elizabeth Margulies, and Abby Nash-Hines from the American Lung Association, Maggie Crawford and Donna O'Neill from Pocket Books, and Megan Gilbert from LifeTime Media for their work on this book. A special thank you to Heather Gautney for her invaluable collaboration in developing initial drafts of this book.

Contents

Preface

by Norman H. Edelman, M.D.,
Scientific Consultant,
The American Lung Association

The American Lung Association is celebrating its hundredth anniversary—that's a century of research and work to prevent lung disease and promote lung health. The Lung Association has saved countless lives and accomplished much, but the battle continues. Lung diseases and breathing problems are the leading causes of infant deaths in the United States today, and asthma is the leading serious chronic childhood illness. Smoking remains the nation's leading preventable cause of death. Lung disease death rates continue to increase while other leading causes of death have declined.

The American Lung Association has long funded vital research on the causes of and treatments for lung disease. It is the foremost defender of the Clean Air Act and laws that protect citizens from secondhand smoke. The Lung Association teaches children the dangers of tobacco use and helps teenage and adult smokers overcome addiction. It educates children and adults living with lung diseases on managing their condition. With the generous support of the public, the American Lung Association is *"Improving life, one breath at a time."*

Through outreach programs and its sponsorship of books like this one, the American Lung Association hopes to encourage people to quit smoking and live healthier, more active lives. In *How to Quit Smoking Without Gaining Weight*, you will learn how to overcome your desire to smoke, how to modify your daily routine to incorporate more physical activity, and how to begin to eat healthier in order to manage your weight. You don't have to put on weight just because you've stopped smoking; with a little help from the American Lung Association, you'll manage cravings by reaching for healthier snacks and replace time once wasted by smoking with physical activity.

The American Lung Association is pleased that Bess Marcus, Jeff Hampl and Ed Fisher joined with us in writing this book. They bring a perfect blend of experience to provide the most up-to-date and comprehensive information on how your efforts to quit smoking can be sidetracked by weight gain and, conversely, how they can be enhanced by physical activity and healthy eating. Dr. Marcus' research on how to help people enjoy greater physical activity has helped many lead healthier lives, including quitting smoking. Dr. Hampl is a leader in turning the complexities of healthy eating into approaches that people can use to live longer and with more energy. Well known for his scholarly work on why people smoke and how they quit, Dr. Fisher has been a volunteer for the American Lung Association for over a quarter century. Together with the American Lung Association, they have developed a book that will help many to quit smoking and lead healthier lives.

For more information about the American Lung Association or to support the work it does, call 1-800-LUNG-USA (1-800-586-4872) or log on to www.lungusa.org.

Facts and Fictions about Quitting Smoking and Managing Your Weight

1

Congratulations! The fact that you opened this book shows that you have taken an interest in quitting smoking and improving your health—and for that alone you deserve a pat on the back! Think it's time to kick the habit? You may feel overwhelmed by the idea or aren't sure that you're ready to do it. Maybe you have even tried to quit before but found it to be too hard and decided not to. Whether you're a first-time quitter or a seasoned veteran, quitting smoking is not an easy thing to do. For most people, there are plenty of obstacles that get in the way. But rest assured, 44.8 million ex-smokers have shown that it can be done, and we are here to help!

If you are especially concerned about gaining weight when you quit, this book is for you. Fear of weight gain is a common reason why people, especially women, do not even attempt to quit smoking. Although statistics vary, as many as 60 percent of men and 51 percent of women gain weight when they quit; 25 percent of women gain in excess of 15 pounds.

We present several strategies and helpful tips here for getting past the obstacles to quitting smoking and on to a healthier way of life—*without expanding your waistline*. Even if you aren't ready to quit yet, focusing on improving other parts of your life, like becoming more physically active or making healthier food choices, can bring you closer to that goal. If you have tried to quit before, we will help you use your past experience to find ways to quit that better fit your lifestyle—so that you can stay smoke-free for good.

Many people think that quitting smoking is either something you can or cannot do. This way of thinking makes the thought of quitting smoking, becoming more physically active, and eating healthier seem like a major test of character. But quitting is not an "all-or-nothing" undertaking. It's really about learning how to make healthy choices—*one day and one choice at a time*. This book will teach you a variety of skills and specific strategies for dealing with difficult situations that test your commitment to quitting, like the urge to smoke a cigarette with your morning coffee or after a meal. Quitting smoking is the result of many individual choices.

Many of the techniques in this book are based on the American Lung Association's Freedom From Smoking® Program and its comprehensive guide to quitting smoking, *7 Steps to a Smoke-Free Life* (1998, LifeTime Media, Inc., Published by John Wiley & Sons, Inc.). We combine the wisdom of American Lung Association programs with our own research on smoking, physical activity, and eating habits, and years of firsthand clinical experience. We have helped thousands of people like you quit smoking and improve their health, and we will provide you with many proven methods for doing the same.

Based on our research and experience, we see quitting smoking, physical activity, and healthy eating as a system of habits that are essential to the overall picture of your health. By working on any one of these elements, it will become easier to make changes in the others. Nicotine is a highly addictive drug, and combined with the habitual nature of smoking, quitting can be a difficult thing to do. Many people use unhealthy foods as a replacement for their smoking habit and as a way of coping with cravings for nicotine. This is part of the reason why smokers tend to gain weight when they quit. We want to help you form new, healthier habits. This means replacing your cigarette addiction with a different kind of "addiction"—satisfying that feeling of wanting something in your mouth by eating some fresh strawberries or carrot sticks. Or by getting addicted to your new aerobics class or a daily walk around the block. Ever notice that people who exercise regularly say they can't live without it? The key is to find physical activities that fit into your lifestyle and healthy foods that satisfy your hunger and taste good. We'll provide you with a firm plan for eating healthier foods and getting more physically active so you can overcome your addiction to smoking and formulate new habits that will keep you healthy and trim.

Timing is key to this process. This book is organized around the physical and psychological changes you may experience over time when you try to quit smoking and manage your weight. This schedule is not set in stone. It is a structure that can help you more easily track your progress and plan your next steps. For example, if you get stuck at any point, you can go back to an earlier lesson and reinforce what you have learned. This happens to most people, so please don't be hard on yourself if it happens to you. The idea is to create and follow a program that you will stick to—one that fits with your routines, but also one that will get you to break some of your not-so-healthy habits and adopt healthier new ones.

Before we move into the core of the program, there are some basic facts about smoking and weight management that you should know. Knowing the basics may help to settle your fears about quitting. In the following pages, we will help you better understand the relationship between smoking and weight gain, and how quitting may affect you physically and emotionally. This information can help prepare you to make decisions about how and when you want to begin the program. Beginning with the facts, the information in this book will supply you with a broad array of tools for becoming a healthier and more energetic person overall.

Introduction to Smoking and Weight Management

The Facts about Quitting and Weight Gain

Quitting smoking is a really tough thing to do, and many people decide not to quit because they are afraid they'll gain weight. You may have tried to quit before and gone back to smoking because you gained five or ten pounds. If these scenarios sound familiar, you are not alone. Many people experience the same anxiety when trying to quit: People gain an average of 10 to 13 pounds when they stop smoking, and many of them return to smoking to lose that weight. This is especially true for women. Experts have found that fear of weight gain is a significant barrier for women who want to quit, and some studies show that women are more likely than men to recognize that they use smoking as a weight-loss strategy. Women are four times more likely than male smokers to report fear of weight gain as a reason for starting to smoke again. Fear can be an obstacle for anyone trying to quit smoking, but it is also one that can be resolved. Just keep the many rewards of quitting in mind: you won't smell of tobacco, you won't be forced to excuse yourself from social situations to smoke a cigarette, you will feel confident and in control. You'll be on the road to looking and feeling more healthy and vibrant! And within a couple of weeks to a month, you will have decreased your chances of heart attack and stroke, you'll breathe easier, your eyes and throat will be less prone to irritation, and walking and other forms of physical activity will get easier. Don't be afraid of living a healthy and smoke-free life!

This is not to say that weight gain is not a real problem for people trying to quit smoking. Keep in mind that some people actually lose weight when they quit smoking, mostly because they make other healthy lifestyle changes in the process, such as becoming more physically active and eating healthier foods. One study, however, showed that major weight gain (roughly 30 pounds or more) occurs in almost 10 percent of men and a little more than 13 percent of women who quit smoking. The risk of being a "supergainer" is greater among those who smoke more than 15 cigarettes per day. People who smoke almost a pack or more a day may want to pay special attention to managing their weight when they quit. But those who smoke at this rate or more are also at higher risk for other negative health effects of smoking.

Regardless of your level of risk, don't let these numbers discourage you or prevent you from attaining your goal. Millions of people have quit successfully and many of them have done so while keeping weight gain to a minimum. It can be done! **Just keep reminding yourself that the strain on your heart from smoking a pack a day is like carrying around 75 to 100 extra pounds of body weight. And, quitting can add 5 to 10 years to your life.** To help you reach your goal, we have designed a program that will help you stay motivated and make use of easy, hassle-free ways to achieve your objectives. Rather than taking a rigid approach to quitting, we believe that a solid, flexible plan that leaves room for the ups and downs of daily life will keep you on track toward a more healthy and smoke-free life.

Quitting and Weight Gain: A Vicious Cycle

When smokers try to quit there are many factors at play, and weight gain is one of them. Pressures to be thin are indeed very strong, and cigarette companies don't make it any easier. They like to play on your desire to be thin, especially if you are a woman. Ads present smoking as a way of controlling weight and coping with life's pressures. Why do you think advertisers tell us that "You've come a long way, baby" and call the product "Virginia Slims"?

Many people get trapped in a vicious cycle of quitting smoking, gaining weight, and going back to smoking. But this merry-go-round of quitting and smoking again doesn't work. Most of the time people do not end up taking off all the weight they gained in the first place, and so they are still smoking cigarettes and endangering their health. Plus smokers then feel frustrated and angry with themselves for failing. This makes it even harder for them to get motivated to make the next attempt to quit.

The best way to get off the merry-go-round is to stop using smoking as a means of managing your weight. This book offers you alternatives that take into account your desire to quit and manage your weight, safely and successfully. Remember, it can and has been done by millions. Like many of those who have quit smoking successfully, you may gain some weight at first. But if you stick with the suggestions in this book, you can avoid or minimize weight gain from the start. In our work, we have found that women who participated in a program of regular physical activity while quitting smoking gained an average of 6 pounds during a 12-week program. Those who were not in the physical activity program gained about 12 pounds. We will provide you with proven methods to minimize weight gain. These may be adapted to your lifestyle so that over the long run—in about a year or so—you can lose any weight you may have gained while quitting smoking and look and feel terrific.

Why People Gain Weight When Quitting

Changes in Metabolism

Scientists have found that smokers generally weigh less than nonsmokers. Smoking may affect the amount and the types of food that people eat and how their body processes food, causing smokers to have a lower body weight. One of the physical reasons some people gain weight when they quit is because of changes in *metabolism*. Your metabolic rate is related to how your body burns calories. It regulates the processes by which your body gets its energy from food, which is vital to its overall function.

Smoking speeds up your metabolism. Here's how it works: Nicotine, just one of the more than 4,000 chemicals in cigarettes, stimulates the central nervous system and other organs. In doing so, it increases the amount of energy you use up. Smoking increases your metabolic rate, so that you burn more calories. When you quit, your metabolic rate slows down to what it was before you started to smoke. For the typical smoker trying to quit, changes in metabolism may result in a weight gain of 2 or 3 pounds. However, it is the increase in eating, particularly foods high in fat or sugar, that results in most of the weight gain that people experience. The good news is that we can help you with your physical activity and food choices to avoid or minimize this kind of weight gain.

One of the most effective ways to manage your weight after quitting is to increase your level of physical activity. Exercise increases metabolism, and even moderate levels of activity can help you burn fat and improve your overall health. Exercise also improves mood, so increases in physical activity such as walking, swimming, doing yard work or even taking the stairs instead of the elevator in your workplace can help you stay positive and assist you in the quitting process. Often raising your level of activity can make a real difference. For example, one study we conducted showed that participating in a regular physical activity program reduced weight gain after quitting and actually increased the chances of quitting successfully. Another study showed that women who report little recreational physical activity have a greater chance of gaining weight after quitting than more active women do.

Later, in chapter five, we will give you specific tips on how to transform some of your daily activities into ways that will raise your metabolic rate. This is something you can work on before, during, and after you start to quit. Making small adjustments in your lifestyle will accelerate your progress toward your goal of better health, a longer life, and more energy to enjoy it. As we said before, timing is an important part of this program. We will help you decide the right time to increase the level of physical activity in your routine. Our goal is to leave you with a sustainable program that is enjoyable, results-oriented, and most important, realistic. This way, physical activity can more easily become a part of your daily life and help keep you healthy and smoke-free. We have already helped thousands of people rediscover the wonders of an active life and we can help you too.

Changes in Eating Style

Healthy eating habits play a key role in maintaining your weight or minimizing weight gain when you quit smoking. Sometimes people gain weight after quitting because of poor eating choices. That is, they simply eat more food, or eat foods that have a lot of fat or sugar. Without the foul taste of cigarettes in your mouth, food may taste and smell better, which could lead to extra helpings at the dinner table. You may also be prone to eating more between meals. Snacking can easily become a substitute for smoking or a way of coping with cravings or stress. Current research indicates that while quitting, many smokers develop cravings for sweet foods, which may be high in calories, fat, and sugar. In fact, some scientists think that nicotine affects the level of blood sugar in the body so that nicotine withdrawal triggers an increased craving for sweet foods. In chapter six, we will talk about how you can substitute tasty and healthy snacks when you are craving a cigarette. We will also give you some tips on how to combat cravings—as well as oral fixation and boredom—by making better food choices. This includes learning how to eat in moderation and how to eat a variety of healthy foods that will give your body the fuel it needs. You may find that within two to three weeks after you stop smoking, the sharpest nicotine cravings will fade and you will have already started to develop healthy eating habits that can benefit you for the rest of your life.

Later in the book, we will cover how you can use healthy snacks and beverages to battle the urge to smoke. Just like smoking, eating is a habit too; no doubt you've become accustomed to eating certain foods. Some foods (chocolate, for example) are high in fat, sugar, and calories. Do you have to give up chocolate for the rest of your life? No! But we want to make sure that you're well aware of the foods you eat and the beverages you drink so that your calories don't creep up during the day. There are no forbidden foods in a healthy eating plan, but some foods you will want to eat often, while others should be saved for special occasions. With this plan, there are no fads, crash diets, or fancy gourmet meals that take hours to prepare. Just sound, nutritional advice to help you quit smoking and manage your weight in the process.

The Dangers of Smoking

A Matter of Life and Death

Now you might be saying to yourself, "Why do they want to tell me this stuff? I already know that smoking is bad for me. Otherwise, I wouldn't have bought this book!" That's true. Most people know that smoking is bad for them. But surveys by the American Lung Association and other health and research organizations show that most people don't realize how *enormously bad* smoking is for them. Doctors are used to patients who say, "Well, I've got to have one vice and other than smoking, I live a pretty healthy life." The fact is, that if you could do only *one* thing to protect your health, not smoking should be No. 1. Recognizing this will help you stay on track when gaining a few pounds might lead you to think you should go back to smoking to shed the weight. That's why we want to review some of the major reasons quitting is the most important thing you can do for yourself.

Smoking is *much* more dangerous to your health than any weight you may gain. This cannot be emphasized enough.

Here are just some of the facts:

- Research shows that about half of all regular cigarette smokers die of smoking-related diseases.

- Smoking is responsible for one in five deaths in the United States.

- More Americans die each year from smoking-related diseases than from AIDS, drug abuse, car accidents, and murder—combined.

- Smoking is directly responsible for 87 percent of lung cancer cases and causes most cases of emphysema and chronic bronchitis.

- Smoking kills more people from coronary heart disease every year than from cancer. Cigarette smoking is a significant risk factor for coronary heart disease. Smoking increases blood pressure, decreases exercise tolerance, and increases the tendency for blood to clot. The U.S. Surgeon General called cigarette smoking "the most important of the known modifiable risk factors for coronary heart disease in the United States."

- Smoking is also a major factor in stroke, and has been linked to a variety of other conditions and disorders, including slowed healing of wounds and infertility.

- Because it causes problems with blood flow, smoking can cause impotence among men.

Smoking is not only bad for your health, but it also harms the environment and endangers the health of those around you. Cigarettes contain at least 69 different chemicals that have been linked to cancer. Every time someone smokes, poisons are released into the air. This means that not only are smokers

Women and Smoking

- Approximately one in five—about 22 million—American women are smokers. Current female smokers aged 35 years or older are 12 times more likely to die prematurely from lung cancer than nonsmoking females.
- Smoking can shave almost 15 years off a woman's life.
- Lung cancer has surpassed breast cancer as the leading cause of cancer deaths among women.
- Smoking during pregnancy accounts for an estimated 20 to 30 percent of low-birth-weight babies, up to 14 percent of pre-term deliveries, and some 10 percent of all infant deaths.

Men and Smoking

- Cigarette smoking is the number one cause of lung cancer death among men.
- Male smokers are almost 10 times more likely to die of bronchitis and emphysema and 22 times more likely to die from lung cancer than non-smoking males.
- Smoking can shave 13 years off a man's life.
- Because of its effects on blood flow, smoking is a major contributor to impotence, especially in men with diabetes or other problems that contribute to impotence.

inhaling these harmful substances, so is everyone else around them. Many studies have shown that secondhand smoke is harmful to nonsmokers and can cause them to develop serious illnesses such as lung and other cancers and coronary heart disease. We know that smoking in the household makes children's asthma worse, and can lead to increased emergency room visits or hospitalizations for asthmatic children. In this light, quitting is especially important for people with children or those planning to have them. Children's lungs are particularly sensitive to their environments and exposure to cigarette smoke early in life can affect lung development and increase the risk for lung disease.

A WORD ABOUT SECONDHAND SMOKE
Secondhand smoke inhaled by nonsmokers from other people's cigarettes is classified by the U.S. Environmental Protection Agency as a known cancer-causing agent, responsible for approximately 3,000 lung cancer deaths each year in U.S. nonsmokers. Don't give your kids or grandkids the "gift" of lung cancer just because you have to smoke.

Nicotine and Addiction

One of the reasons why it is so hard to quit smoking is because of the presence of nicotine in cigarettes. Nicotine is an addictive drug. In fact, the Surgeon General has reported that cigarettes are just as addictive as cocaine or heroin.

Nicotine can have different effects at different times, and most experienced smokers are pretty good at getting all of them. It can act as an "upper" and speed up many body reactions. Or it can act as a "downer" and reduce anxiety. How it works depends on several factors—the amount of nicotine in the body, the time passed since the last cigarette, stress level, and time of day. Early in the day nicotine acts as a stimulant to many people. Later in the day it seems to act more as a sedative and helps people to relax. Nicotine also raises mood—in this way, it helps smokers cope with low moods or sadness.

The fact that smoking may raise one's mood, reduce anxiety, and even increase alertness makes it all the more attractive. That's why people who are under stress or feel nervous or bored often are at greater risk of becoming addicted to nicotine. What may be the most troublesome part of all of this is the fact that cigarettes are ideal ways of getting nicotine to people. It only takes 7 seconds from the time you inhale to the time nicotine hits your brain. That's why that first puff after a long movie feels so good—7 seconds and nirvana, here I come! Physical activity is a great substitute for smoking in this regard. With it, you can reduce tension, raise your mood and help fight depression and anxiety without putting your health and well being at risk. We'll go over this in chapter five.

The habitual nature of smoking also contributes to the difficulty of quitting. Smokers get hooked on the taste, smell, and feel of cigarettes. They link smoking with many activities. Some people like to smoke when they are talking on the telephone or having a cup of coffee. Other people like to smoke at parties or when they are relaxing at home. The person who has smoked a pack a day for 20 years—maybe you—has inhaled over a million times (7 puffs per cigarette x 20 cigarettes a day x 365 days a year x 20 years = 1,022,000). The combination of nicotine addiction and these kinds of strong mental links makes smoking a tough habit to break.

Smoking is used by many people as a way of coping with life's pressures, and nicotine withdrawal can increase your anxiety and stress. After quitting, many people turn to food to relieve feelings of anxiety and develop unhealthy eating habits. By coupling quitting smoking with eating balanced meals and healthy snacks, you can start to break the links between feelings of anxiety and use of both foods and cigarettes for comfort. Walking and other forms of physical activity can relieve stress, can help you sleep better, and can have an overall calming effect. And, in addition to physical activity and making healthy eating choices, there is a broad range of techniques to help you quit, including nicotine replacement, other medicines, and group smoking cessation programs to help you. There are plenty of ways to learn to cope with stress or boredom besides nicotine. We will review these many options and help tailor them to meet your specific needs.

!

SMOKING CAN MAKE YOU LOOK BAD

Smoking is bad for the way you look. Quitting may mean weight gain, but smoking is almost certain to yellow your teeth, stain your fingers, and result in bad breath. Smoking also affects your complexion. It is a main cause of premature aging of the skin, as evidenced by wrinkles.

The Personal and Social Costs of Smoking

Smoking can negatively affect your appearance, but there are other costs as well, including social isolation. Increasing public sentiment against smoking combined with knowledge of the effects of secondhand smoke have influenced public policy to the extent that many cities around the country such as Boston, New York, San Francisco, and Anchorage have banned smoking in most public places, including office buildings, bars, and restaurants. People who smoke now have to stand outside to get their fix. In addition, many states have instituted high taxes on cigarettes in an attempt to discourage smoking, thereby increasing the cost of that nicotine. For example, a pack a day in many states costs roughly $2,500 per year—more than enough for a health club membership and maybe even a personal trainer or a great vacation. The American Lung Association's *State of Tobacco Control: 2003* is a great resource for finding out about the tobacco control laws in your state. It can be accessed via the American Lung Association's website at www.lungusa.org under "tobacco control." The site also provides information about new research on state tobacco laws, which has shown that high taxes and bans have indeed been effective in getting people to quit smoking. Despite the fact that fewer people are smoking, the cost to society is still very high. Smoking costs the nation over $150 billion per year in health care costs and lost productivity from missing days at work. Personally, it could cost you your life—which is why we want to help you quit today!

Quitting Smoking + Physical Activity + Healthy Eating = A Healthy New You

The good news: there are ways to quit smoking and stay smoke-free. Making healthy food choices and incorporating physical activity in your daily routines are central themes with us because they can help you avoid gaining weight or minimize the amount of weight you gain. They are also a vital part of developing a healthy lifestyle. Physical activity and healthy eating go hand in hand and are well-known ways to prevent cancer and coronary heart disease, the primary causes of death in the United States. Physical activity and healthy eating reinforce each other, and can also reinforce your decision to quit. Within a year of quitting you will reduce your chances of getting heart disease by as much as half. But the way in which you quit—by using physical activity and healthy eating to help you in the process—also significantly lowers health risks, including heart disease.

We understand that quitting is a difficult process and that it takes time. If you aren't quite ready, we will help you get there and we hope you are proud of yourself for opening this book and reading this far. This is a huge step forward in the likelihood that you will one day be an ex-smoker.

Healthy Living 101

2

Welcome to "Healthy Living 101." Like an introductory "101" class, this chapter will familiarize you with key concepts for working on your health in the core areas of quitting smoking, physical activity, and healthy eating. Now that you've completed chapter one and better understand the basics of quitting smoking and managing your weight, we can build on that knowledge to prepare you for what to expect and how to do it smoothly and effectively.

As you build a healthy lifestyle, you can expect to experience some positive changes in your general appearance. People who eat well and are regularly active tend to have a bright, healthy outlook and more energy to live life to the fullest. They also tend to weigh less. Exercise is a proven way to lose weight and become physically fit, which means more flexibility, a higher level of endurance, better muscle tone, and stronger bones and joints. Combined with a healthy eating plan, it can help keep you feeling healthy, trim, and perhaps best of all, help you stay away from cigarettes.

We mentioned earlier that the nicotine in cigarettes is

highly addictive. Even if you haven't developed a physical addiction, smoking may have become a regular behavior, or habit, in your daily life. The combination of the physical addiction to nicotine in cigarettes and the habit of smoking can make quitting extremely difficult. In this chapter, we'll show you how to overcome your addiction to cigarettes and your smoking habit while building a healthier lifestyle overall. As the box below shows, physical activity and healthy eating are key to this process—they work together to help you quit and manage your weight.

How Quitting, Physical Activity, and Making Healthy Eating Choices Work Together

- Eating healthy foods can make quitting smoking easier. Making healthy eating choices can also reduce the amount of weight you may gain.
- Physical activity helps to reduce stress so that you feel more relaxed and alert.
- Physical activity can increase the rate at which your body burns calories and help you lose fat while gaining muscle tone.
- Managing your life in any one of these ways will help boost your self-esteem and help you to feel more in control of your life.
- Physical activity and a healthy diet can lift your mood and keep you feeling energized and in control.
- Cigarette smoking is a major risk factor for coronary heart disease. Physical activity and healthy eating are proven ways for reducing risks associated with heart disease and even reversing some of smoking's harmful effects.

Getting Started 101

Looking at Your Habits

Just because quitting smoking, physical activity, and healthy eating work so well together does not mean that you must focus on all of these areas at once. And even if you do, you are bound to move faster in one area than in the others. Think of it more as a chain reaction. Breaking your smoking habit should be your number-one priority, but this is not an all-or-nothing process. By making healthy lifestyle choices in one of these areas, you will set yourself in motion for making positive changes in the others.

This book was designed to accommodate your particular pace. It works by first giving you a sound method for quitting smoking and managing your weight. But we also want you to *stay* smoke-free and manage your weight over the years. In our experience, focusing on your daily routines is one of the best ways to ensure that the changes you make now will continue over time. This means breaking some of the habits that jeopardize your health and replacing them with new, healthy ones.

These lifelong lessons can be applied to many different parts of your life. Think of things that you may have changed successfully in the past. Maybe you tried to use less salt when you cooked and found new ways of making bland foods taste better by using different spices or methods of preparation. Maybe you wanted to watch less TV and started reading more. In the following exercise, make a list of habits in your life that you have changed for the better. Reflect for a moment on what helped you succeed and what got in the way.

When you think about it, there are probably many positive changes you have made in your life. Quitting smoking and managing your weight work the same way—and can be

ASSIGNMENT:
Looking at Your Habits

HABITS I'VE CHANGED

1.

2.

3.

THINGS THAT HELPED ME SUCCEED

1.

2.

3.

OBSTACLES THAT GOT IN THE WAY

1.

2.

3.

Reprinted, by permission, from B.H. Marcus & L.H. Forsyth, 2003, *Motivating people to be physically active* (Champaign, IL: Human Kinetics), 134.

another one of your success stories. Remember, you should feel proud of yourself for making the difficult decision to quit smoking. Now all you need is a solid plan for accomplishing your goal of living a healthy, smoke-free life.

Planning Ahead for Your New Smoke-Free Life

Just like using a road map to plan a trip or making blueprints before building a house, planning can go a long way in making sure you don't lose sight of your goal. Making changes that affect your daily routine requires some planning, and planning can get you psyched about the process of building a healthy life. You may have already tried to quit, but couldn't get past the craving for an after-dinner cigarette. Or maybe you've tried to start being more physically active, but simply couldn't find the time. We can show you how to get past these kinds of barriers by planning ahead and finding ways to fit a brisk walk into your day—maybe even after dinner when you feel the temptation to smoke.

Planning ahead includes a close look at your reasons for wanting to make certain changes in your life. You may be concerned about your health and the dangers of smoking but are worried that you will gain weight if you quit. You may want to eat more balanced meals, but think they will take too much time to prepare. The process of identifying your reasons for wanting to change can help you see the difference between the things you can control and those you cannot. Sometimes, the biggest obstacle to any kind of change is self-doubt—worrying about how hard it may be or making excuses for why it can't happen now. Realizing your reasons for wanting to make changes in your life may be what convinces you to stop smoking and make other healthy decisions. And if you're not sure how to begin to change your routine, we will take you through some exercises that can help get you on the right track.

Planning ahead also means looking at parts of your everyday life that might make it difficult to stop smoking. Habits become part of our daily routines and many times we don't even realize we've developed them, which makes them difficult to break. The solution is to first recognize them. Understanding your eating habits—for example, knowing when you tend to overeat and how you feel when you do—can highlight opportunities for change. Being aware of the obstacles in your daily life will help you find ways around them or replace them with healthier choices. For example, you can cope with cigarette cravings by eating healthy snack foods, such as fruit popsicles, graham crackers, or low-fat yogurts. The next time you are tempted to devour a bag of potato chips, you can decide ahead of time that you will stop and take a brisk walk before eating even one chip. In all likelihood you won't go back to the chips because the craving will have passed. Managing your cravings is an important element of quitting smoking, and you can do it—as long as you plan ahead.

Barriers can also be overcome by simply removing temptations from your physical environment. Getting rid of the cigarettes and ashtrays in your home or office is an absolute must for avoiding the temptation to smoke. If you want to start increasing your level of physical activity, clear a corner of the living room where you can stretch, do breathing exercises or put that exercise equipment that has been gathering dust in the basement. Friends, family and co-workers can also help get you through the tough times, even those who are not very supportive at first. Start by informing everyone you know that you want to quit. People who don't smoke will be happy to hear it and the smokers in your life will likely respect your choice. They may even want to try it themselves.

Planning healthy meals with friends, taking a yoga or dance class, playing soccer with the kids are all ways that you can fill the time you may have spent smoking with fun activities that are also good for your health. A nurturing and supportive environment is a valuable asset when trying to make tough changes. In chapter six, we'll give you some advice on how to gain the support of your friends and family if you aren't sure where to begin.

In the next chapter, we will go further into the process of identifying your obstacles to success and providing simple, practical tips for how to get past them. Rewards are a big part of the plan and give you something to look forward to. Each time you get past a hurdle or reach a milestone, celebrate your success by buying that new pair of shoes you always wanted, going out to the movies, or letting yourself sleep in for a change.

Quitting Smoking 101

"One day I was walking up the stairs to my apartment and I was out of breath. It was scary. The first thing I thought was, I've got to quit smoking. I decided to try quitting. Well, it wasn't a snap. But taking it a step at a time worked and you wouldn't believe it: a few weeks later I was practically running up those stairs!" (Charles, age 53)

The Benefits of Quitting

Smoking cigarettes can make even simple, everyday tasks difficult. Indeed, smoking carries a high cost—not only to your wallet, but more important, to your health. You probably know that quitting is a tough thing to do, but you may not realize how much better you will feel and how soon. Within weeks after you quit smoking:

- Your appearance will improve—no more cigarette breath or tobacco-stained hands, and you won't be damaging your skin further. Remember, smoking causes wrinkles!

- You will have more energy.

- Your eyes and throat will be less prone to irritation.

- Your smoker's cough will go away.

- Your senses of taste and smell will become more acute.

- You'll have fewer colds and bouts of the flu.

Some Additional Benefits of Quitting

- You will have more stamina for exercise.
- You will have more money to spend.
- Your circulation will improve.
- You won't smell of tobacco.
- If you smoke at home, you will reduce the risk of fire hazard.
- If you are pregnant, you will reduce health risks for your unborn child.
- Your life won't be controlled by addiction to cigarettes.

These benefits increase over time. As your body starts to repair some of the damage done by smoking, you significantly lower your risk for coronary heart disease, cancer, high blood pressure, emphysema, and a whole host of other threats to your health.

Short and Long Term Health Benefits of Quitting Smoking

20 MINUTES AFTER YOUR LAST CIGARETTE

- blood pressure drops to normal
- pulse rate drops to normal
- body temperature of hands and feet increases to normal

8 HOURS

- carbon monoxide level in blood returns to normal
- oxygen level in blood increases to normal

24 HOURS

- chance of a heart attack decreases

48 HOURS

- ability to smell and taste is enhanced

2 WEEKS TO 3 MONTHS

- circulation improves
- walking becomes easier
- lung function increases

1 TO 9 MONTHS

- coughing, sinus congestion, fatigue, shortness of breath decrease

AT 1 YEAR

- excess risk of coronary heart disease is decreased to half that of a smoker

AT 5 YEARS

- risk of cancer of the mouth, throat, and esophagus is halved compared to non-smokers
- 5 to 15 years after quitting, stroke risk is reduced to that of people who have never smoked

AT 10 YEARS

- risk of lung cancer drops to as little as half that of continuing smokers
- risk of cancer of the larynx, bladder, kidney, and pancreas decreases
- risk of ulcer decreases

AT 15 YEARS

- risk of coronary heart disease is now similar to that of people who have never smoked
- risk of death returns to nearly the level of people who have never smoked

Smoking and Addiction

Now you might be thinking, "Quitting smoking may be good for me, but it's not easy to do." You're absolutely right. Most people who smoke know that it is bad for their health and are well aware of the many good reasons they should quit. But knowing doesn't make it any easier to break the habit.

As we mentioned earlier, the reason why it's so hard to quit is that smoking is *both* a habit and an addiction. Most people who have had trouble quitting are addicted to the nicotine in cigarettes. And the fact that smoking is tied to so many activities in our daily lives makes the addiction to smoking more powerful.

If your body has become accustomed to having its nicotine, you may experience withdrawal symptoms when you quit, such as changes in your mood and energy level. But quitting can affect people in different ways. Some people report being very sleepy and having difficulty concentrating, while others say they

How Addicted Are You?

ASK YOURSELF THE FOLLOWING QUESTIONS
- Do you smoke your first cigarette within 30 minutes of waking up?
- Do you smoke a pack or more per day?
- Do you crave cigarettes in situations where you can't have one or don't have any left?
- Is it tough to keep from smoking for more than just a few hours?
- When you are sick enough to stay in bed, do you still smoke?

If you answered yes to two or more of these questions, you are probably addicted to nicotine and may want to think seriously about strengthening your efforts to quit by using nicotine gum or nicotine patches or by talking to your doctor about Zyban® or other medications for which you need a prescription.

feel nervous and irritable. Still others report feeling intense cravings for tobacco or sweets, or having terrible headaches.

Although you may experience any or all of these symptoms, the good news is that they don't last forever. Studies show that although depression, anxiety, irritability, anger, and fatigue are symptoms that have been reported by people after they quit, these symptoms tend to peak within a few days of quitting and then go away. Healthy eating and physical activity can help alleviate these symptoms. A well-balanced diet and increased physical activity can give you the energy you need to get through the day. Physical activity is a natural, healthy way to help manage stress, anxiety, and low mood. It can also help you to fill in the now-empty spaces that cigarettes may have occupied in your life. This is why we suggest that you start thinking about your eating habits and becoming more physically active *before* you try to quit. It can make quitting easier and can help you manage your weight.

Remember, the American Lung Association has helped thousands of people kick the habit over the years and one of those can—and should—be you! You don't have to quit "cold turkey"—there are other methods available now to help you deal with nicotine withdrawal.

Nicotine patches or nicotine gum found in a pharmacy and new prescription medications can help to reduce cravings for nicotine so that you can focus on habit change. The charts on the following pages can help you decide which one is right for you.

Part of preparing to quit is finding ways that fit your lifestyle, your needs, and your smoking habit. There is no "right way" to quit. If one method is not for you, there are plenty of other choices available. The "right way" is the way that works for you.

A Word about Smokeless Tobacco

Smokeless tobacco, sometimes called "snuff" or "chew," should NOT be used as a substitute for smoking. Because smokeless tobacco contains many of the same chemicals as cigarettes, it causes many of the same negative health effects associated with smoking. These include cancers, including those of the mouth and jaw, bad breath, numbing of the taste buds, and stained teeth. Smokeless tobacco is kept in your mouth and using it can lead to gum disease and tooth loss. All forms of tobacco are bad for you. If you really want to chew on something, try nicotine gum, sugarless gum, or some healthy snacks, such as low-fat fruit or fig bars, flavored rice cakes, or the many others listed on pages 81-83.

Don't confuse nicotine gum with smokeless tobacco. Although too much nicotine can cause some problems, it's not the nicotine in cigarettes that kills people, but all the other chemicals that go along with it. And smokeless tobacco includes a lot of these other chemicals too. Nicotine gum has just enough nicotine to help you until the worst is over. It can help you focus on resisting those urges and living a healthy life without nicotine.

Smoking: A Tough Habit to Break

While there are many ways to cope with nicotine addiction, overcoming that addiction is often not the only obstacle to quitting. For many people, smoking is a habit that is attached to a variety of behaviors, some of which they are not even aware.

Many people tend to smoke at specific times during the day or reach for a cigarette in stressful times or when feeling low. The same goes for eating and physical activity. Some people overeat when they are nervous or don't go to the gym because they feel too depressed. In fact, smoking, physical activity, and eating style are often part of the same system of habits.

Group Smoking Cessation Programs

Group smoking cessation programs can be very helpful in providing peer support and experienced counselors to help monitor your progress. The cost of these programs vary from almost nothing to hundreds of dollars, but a higher cost does not necessarily guarantee success. Many health plans and workplaces provide free programs for quitting smoking and some health plans will cover the cost of medications to help you quit. Check with your insurance carrier or employer for more information. In addition, when deciding which program is right for you, consider whether the program is conveniently located, if the staff is well trained and professional, whether the program meets your particular needs, and its success rate. Remember, there are no tricks or magic bullets to make you stop smoking. If a program seems too easy, guarantees that you will quit, or claims to have a success rate that seems unrealistic, you might want to look elsewhere. American Lung Association Freedom From Smoking® (FFS) Cessation Clinics have a proven track record and have helped thousands of people quit smoking over the years. The FFS program consists of eight group sessions, and uses a positive behavior-change approach that teaches the smoker how to quit. It focuses on developing a quitting strategy, understanding nicotine addiction and the use of nicotine replacement products, dealing with recovery symptoms, controlling weight, and managing stress through relaxation, as well as assertiveness techniques and a variety of relapse prevention strategies for staying off cigarettes. Call 1-800-LUNGUSA for the American Lung Association Freedom From Smoking® Cessation Clinic in your area. You can also access the FFS program through Freedom From Smoking® Online at www.ffsonline.org.

Which Nicotine Replacement Product Is Right for Me?

Nicotine Patch

WHAT IT IS

Nicoderm® CQ

Nicotrol®

Habitrol®
(prescription required)

ProStep®
(prescription required)

Patches deliver nicotine through the skin in different strengths, over different lengths of time.

HOW IT'S USED

Patches vary in strength and the length of time they can be used. Depending on the brand you use, the patch may be left on anywhere from 16 to 24 hours.

PROS

- easy to use
- only needs to be applied once a day
- some available without prescription
- few side effects

CONS

- less flexible dosing
- slow onset of delivery
- mild skin rashes and irritation

ADDITIONAL INFORMATION

Some smokers who use these products can stop using them abruptly while others prefer to reduce their dosage slowly.

Adapted from the American Lung Association's "Quit Smoking Action Plan."

Nicotine Polacrilex (nicotine gum)

WHAT IT IS

Nicorette®

The term "gum" is misleading. Although it actually is a gum-like substance with small amounts of nicotine, it is not like regular gum. Instead, you chew briefly and then place it between your cheek and gum. The nicotine is absorbed through the lining of the mouth.

HOW IT'S USED

It is recommended that you chew enough gum to reduce withdrawal symptoms (10–15 pieces a day but no more than 30 a day).

PROS

- convenient
- flexible dosing
- faster delivery of nicotine than the patches

CONS

- may be inappropriate for people with dental problems and those with temporomandibular joint syndrome (TMJ)
- cannot eat or drink while medication is in your mouth
- frequent use during the day is required to obtain adequate nicotine levels

ADDITIONAL INFORMATION

Many people use the medication incorrectly. Most of the time the gum is in your mouth, it should be placed between your cheek and gum. Read package directions carefully for a full explanation.

Which Nicotine Replacement Product Is Right for Me? *Continued*

Nicotine Lozenges

WHAT IT IS
Commit®

HOW IT'S USED
Recommended dosage is at least 9 pieces per day during the first 6 weeks of the 12-week program. Available in 2 mg and 4 mg dosages depending on the timing of when you would have your first cigarette.

PROS
- convenient
- flexible dosing
- faster delivery of nicotine than the patches
- available without a prescription

CONS
- frequent use during the day is required to obtain adequate nicotine levels
- cannot eat or drink while medication is in your mouth

ADDITIONAL INFORMATION
This product is different from nicotine gum as it is meant to be sucked on and moved from side to side in your mouth until it dissolves, like hard candy or a medicinal lozenge.

Nicotine Nasal Spray

WHAT IT IS
Nicotrol® NS
(prescription required)

HOW IT'S USED
Delivers nicotine through the lining of the nose when you squirt it directly into each nostril.

PROS
- flexible dosing
- can be used in response to stress or urges to smoke
- fastest delivery of nicotine of current available products
- reduces cravings within minutes

CONS
- nose and eye irritation is common, but usually disappears within one week
- frequent use during the day is required to obtain adequate nicotine levels

Which Nicotine Replacement Product Is Right for Me? *Continued*

Nicotine Inhaler

WHAT IT IS

Nicotrol® Inhaler (prescription required)

A plastic cylinder containing a cartridge that delivers nicotine when you puff on it.

It looks like a cigarette, but delivers nicotine into the mouth and not the lung.

HOW IT'S USED

Puffing must be done frequently, far more often than your cigarette. Each cartridge lasts for 80 long puffs; each cartridge is designed for 20 minutes of use. A minimum of six cartridges per day is needed for three to six weeks.

PROS
- flexible dosing
- faster delivery of nicotine than the patches
- few side effects
- mimics the hand-to-mouth behavior of smoking

CONS
- frequent use during the day is required to obtain adequate nicotine levels
- may cause mouth or throat irritation

ADDITIONAL INFORMATION

You do not need to inhale deeply to achieve an effect. Small doses of nicotine provide a sensation in the back of the throat similar to cigarette smoke.

Non-Nicotine Medication

WHAT IT IS

Zyban™ (bupropion hydrochloride) Sustained-Release Tablets (prescription required)

Currently the only non-nicotine medication shown to be effective for quitting smoking. Treatment must be started at least one week before your Quit Day.

HOW IT'S USED

The usual dosage is to take two tablets per day.

PROS

- easy to use
- pill form
- few side effects
- can be used in combination with nicotine patches

CONS

- should not be used by patients with eating disorders, seizure disorders or those taking certain other medications
- lack of flexibility of use

ADDITIONAL INFORMATION

This is the first medication to help people quit smoking that is available in tablet form. Its primary role is to act on brain chemistry to bring about some of the same effects that nicotine has when people smoke. A small risk of seizure is associated with use of this medication. The main ingredient in Zyban™ has been available for many years as a treatment for depression under the trade name Wellbutrin. However, it works well as an aid to quit smoking.

The three tend to work off each other and links between certain behaviors can be very strong and difficult to undo. But it is also for this reason that physical activity and healthy eating practices can help you kick your smoking habit.

Here is a classic example: Many smokers like to have a cigarette after a meal. Then, when they quit, they use food as a substitute for smoking and often gain weight as a result. But finding healthier food substitutes, such as an apple or frozen yogurt instead of ice cream after dinner can help you get through the cravings and avoid gaining extra weight. Did you know that smoking can decrease your stamina for physical activity? You may have felt this the last time you tried to go for a jog or climbed a steep set of stairs. But increasing your level of activity in even the simplest ways can build your stamina back up. And believe it or not, being more physically active can also help curb your cigarette cravings.

As health experts, we know of many healthy ways to cope with the stressful effects of quitting smoking and managing your weight. Managing your stress, as well as your down time, can be achieved through relaxation exercises, deep breathing, and of course, physical activity and healthy eating. In the upcoming chapters, we will give you many tips on how to substitute more healthy behaviors for smoking. Think of these as your instruments for an exciting new experiment. Routines can be boring. Here is an opportunity to test different ways of making your daily life more dynamic.

Physical Activity 101

Making a Habit Out of Physical Activity

"I have tried so many times to start an exercise program. Gym memberships, exercise machines... even a karate class. One day my roommate suggested we start taking walks together, just a couple days a week before we start our day. This was usually the time I would have my morning coffee and, of course, a cigarette. I found it much nicer to walk with her and enjoy the morning air. We liked it so much, now we walk every day! Now I have more energy throughout the rest of my day and find myself not even wanting to smoke." (Tracy, age 35)

There are countless benefits to leading an active life and making physical activity a part of your daily routine. Many people find that physical activity is a great way to spend time with their loved ones, and make new friends or discover old ones. For Tracy, what started out as a frustrating situation turned into an opportunity to spend some quality time with her roommate. And, it helped curb her smoking habit. Some people, on the other hand, see their physical activity routine as "me time"—time to relax and be by yourself, away from the hustle and bustle of work and home life.

Increasing your level of physical activity can also lead you to develop new interests. Some people join health clubs or community centers and meet new friends, while others take classes and learn a new skill such as self-defense or cardio kick-boxing. Even activities that don't require much planning can help—such as walking around the airport terminal when you're traveling, instead of sitting outside the gate, waiting. The possibilities are infinite.

Time is one of the most common roadblocks for people

who want to start getting more physically active. But instead of running headfirst into an intense program or an hour-long exercise tape, begin slowly. Start by finding those 5 or 10 minutes where you can transform your everyday activities into opportunities for physical activity. Try to be creative and make it something you enjoy.

If you are concerned about cost, don't worry. Physical activity does not require gym memberships or expensive classes. It can be done in the settings of your daily life—at home and in the office. Some people like to exercise in front of the TV or while listening to music. The great thing about being active in your home is that it's hassle free and you will be setting a great example for the rest of your family. Once they see how great you're doing, they may even want to join you.

As for work, many of us have the type of jobs that keep us in a chair behind a desk all day. Taking the stairs instead of the elevator can raise your heart rate. Even walking to the end of the hall to see a colleague instead of calling or sending an email can be an easy way to get in a little physical activity. In chapter 5, we will help you go through your typical schedule to help you make time for physical activity. We will also give you some handy tips for how to take what you are already doing and use it as a chance to get more active.

The Benefits of Physical Activity

Physical activity is absolutely vital to your overall health and can significantly lower your risk of disease. Organizations like the American Heart Association estimate that about 300,000 deaths per year in the United States are related to poor diet and physical inactivity. Lack of physical activity has been proven to be a risk for serious illnesses, including coronary heart disease, high blood pressure, and stroke. Certain populations—such as

Some Benefits of Physical Activity

- You will feel less stressed.
- Your appearance will brighten as well as your general outlook.
- You will have a tool to manage your weight and even lose some if you want.
- You will have reduced your risk of heart disease, high blood pressure, diabetes, colon cancer, and other diseases.
- Your self-image will likely improve as you begin to get more physically fit.
- You will increase your muscle tone and build stronger bones and joints.
- You will have a longer, healthier life overall.

older adults and those with low incomes—are especially at risk: 65 percent of them are less active than they should be. Physical activity also reduces the risk of colon cancer and builds strong bones, muscles, and joints, and can help people to manage health problems such as diabetes and obesity. Even moderately intense physical activities—such as doing heavy housework or climbing stairs—can help if done regularly.

Physical activity can also increase your chances of successfully kicking your smoking habit. In our studies, women who were physically active while trying to quit were twice as likely to stay off cigarettes than those who did not. We also found that they gained about half the weight of women who were not physically active. In another study, we found that the women who were physically active said they had decreased urges to smoke after their training sessions. By using physical activity as a substitute for smoking you are really doing two things at once —working on physical fitness and filling the time you may have smoked with a more healthy activity. It is also a great chance to socialize. Playing tennis or racquetball with a friend, going

Quitting Smoking and Managing Your Weight: Walking, Cycling, and Swimming Can Help

Walking, cycling, and swimming can help you quit smoking and manage your weight. These activities involve sustained aerobic effort, which can boost your metabolism, burn calories and fat, and help to reduce stress. Swimming and biking are excellent because it's almost impossible to smoke or eat fattening foods while exercising. You don't need expensive equipment to walk, cycle, or swim. Research also suggests that sustained aerobic exercise can help offset nicotine cravings and elevate mood. In chapter five we will discuss how you can integrate a meaningful exercise program into your life using these and other kinds of simple and enjoyable physical activities.

Physical activity can also help you psychologically. It can reduce stress and anxiety and help you sleep better at night. It helps to improve mood and combat depression, especially those low moods associated with quitting smoking. Cigarettes can make you feel more alert. Why not achieve that same feeling of alertness from physical activity instead of from a cigarette? Physical activity can positively affect your self-esteem, including your body image, which can play an important role in smoking behavior. In our research, we found that women who smoked tended to have a poorer body image than those who did not smoke. We concluded that this could be a factor in quitting smoking, as women with a poor body image might be concerned about potential weight gain.

Physical activity can help you manage your weight and become more physically fit, which can improve your body image and make you feel better about yourself. Substituting physical activity for smoking may help you manage cravings and fill time once used to smoke cigarettes. And once you get started, you are likely to find that you have increased energy, a more positive outlook, an overall sense of well-being, and, the knowledge that you are on the way to living a longer, happier life.

dancing at a smoke-free club, or just taking a brisk walk around the mall can provide great opportunities for catching up with friends and getting to know new ones.

Getting Started Safely

Although moderate-intensity activities are generally safe for most people, some people have pre-existing conditions that can affect their ability to be active. Before you start to increase your activity at any level, complete the Physical Activity Readiness Questionnaire (PAR-Q) on page 46. If you answer yes to any of the questions, consult your doctor about the ones that apply to you. Your doctor may give you an exercise stress test to see how much physical activity you should be doing and for how long. If you answer no to all of the questions, you are ready to begin. During the process of starting up and even once you have made physical activity a regular habit, make sure to consult your doctor if you start to experience any of the symptoms in the questionnaire.

If you decide that you want to start right off with vigorous intensity activities, like running or swimming, we recommend that you consult with your doctor if one or more of the following applies to you:

- You are a man 45 or older or a woman 55 or older.

- You have one of the following risk factors for coronary heart disease, in addition to being a smoker: high blood

Physical Activity Readiness Questionnaire (PAR-Q)

Regular physical activity is fun and healthy, and increasingly more people are starting to become more active every day. Being more active is very safe for most people. However, some people should check with their health care provider before they start becoming much more physically active. If you are planning to become much more physically active than you are now, start by answering the seven questions in the box below. If you are between the ages of 15 and 69, the PAR-Q will tell you if you should check with your health care provider before you start. If you are over age 69 and not used to being very active, check with your health care provider. Common sense is your best guide when you answer these questions. Please read the questions carefully and answer each one honestly: check YES or NO.

1 Has your health care provider ever said that you have a heart condition and that you should only do physical activity recommended by a health care provider?   YES ☐   NO ☐

2 Do you feel pain in your chest when you do physical activity?   YES ☐   NO ☐

3 In the past month, have you had chest pain when you were not doing physical activity?   YES ☐   NO ☐

4 Do you lose your balance because of dizziness or do you ever lose consciousness?   YES ☐   NO ☐

5 Do you have a bone or joint problem that could be made worse by a change in your physical activity?   YES ☐   NO ☐

6 Is your health care provider currently prescribing drugs (for example, water pills) for your blood pressure or heart condition?   YES ☐   NO ☐

7 Do you know of any other reason why you should not exercise?   YES ☐   NO ☐

Source: Physical Activity Readiness Questionnaire (PAR-Q) © 2002. Reprinted with permission from the Canadian Society for Exercise Physiology. www.csep.ca/forms.asp.

pressure, high cholesterol, high blood sugar, 30 pounds or more overweight, currently not at all active, family history of heart disease.

- ◆ You have heart or blood vessel disease, diabetes, lung disease, asthma, thyroid disorder, or kidney disease.

Adapted from B.H. Marcus and L.H. Forsyth, *Motivating People to Be Physically Active* (Champaign, IL: Human Kinetics, 2003).

Healthy Eating Habits 101

"I have tried so many diets and none of them worked. Most diets required that I starve myself or eat foods that tasted terrible. I also noticed that when I tried to diet, I smoked a lot more. Now, I am trying to take a little more time with my eating. Instead of rushing around, I am thinking more about what I eat and when—and also, trying to count to ten before I reach for that cigarette." (Carmen, age 38)

Eating Well

Earlier in this chapter, we talked about quitting smoking and becoming physically active. Now we turn to the third component of your new healthy lifestyle—healthy eating. You may have noticed that we don't use the word "diet" in this book. That's because when people hear the D word, they usually stop listening. Healthy eating isn't about dieting. Dieting is short-term, a quick fix. Eating well isn't something you do for a week or two. We want you to focus on eating well for the rest of your life. Of course, some of you may feel a bit overwhelmed by all this talk of "the rest of your life." You may be thinking, "Hey, I just wanted to quit smoking without putting on some extra pounds, not get a health make-over." Don't worry too much about this, because what we're talking about here is not converting you to marathon training and an all-seaweed diet. Just making moderate changes in your physical activity and eating habits will add up to big health benefits, in addition to helping you quit smoking.

The Wisdom of the Pyramid

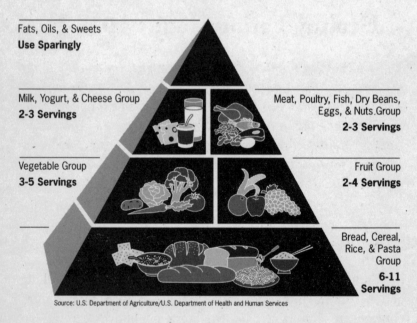

Fats, Oils, & Sweets
Use Sparingly

Milk, Yogurt, & Cheese Group
2-3 Servings

Meat, Poultry, Fish, Dry Beans, Eggs, & Nuts Group
2-3 Servings

Vegetable Group
3-5 Servings

Fruit Group
2-4 Servings

Bread, Cereal, Rice, & Pasta Group
6-11 Servings

Source: U.S. Department of Agriculture/U.S. Department of Health and Human Services

You've probably seen the Food Guide Pyramid on food labels or posters before. Take a minute to look at the Pyramid and how many servings you should have from each section.

The base of the Pyramid is called "bread, cereals, rice, and pasta," and you should have six to eleven servings of these each day. Yes, that does sound like a *lot* of food, but, chances are, you're already probably eating that much. A serving is one slice of bread, one ounce of ready-to-eat cereal, or a half cup of cooked rice or pasta. Think back to the last time you had spaghetti. How many servings did you have? You probably had more than just a half cup. Over the years, our servings sizes in the United States have grown. For example, the bagel you bought at the coffee shop on your way to work probably represented three servings from the Pyramid because of its size.

You might be saying to yourself, "Do I have to measure my food every time I want to eat?" The answer is no. Establishing a nutritious eating style does not have to be a painstaking experience, but you will need a little practice before you get the hang of it. Take a couple of days when you aren't too busy or stressed, and try measuring your food portions to get a feel for what a serving size looks like. Most food labels contain serving size information on the nutrition label, but for some foods, such as pizza, you will need to estimate. It's much easier than it sounds. Next time you are ready to make a pasta salad, simply take out a measuring cup and use it to get a good estimate of the serving size. As we said above, half a cup of pasta is equal to one serving. For items such as cheeses and meats, you will need to weigh the item to determine its serving size. Small scales that measure ounces are available in most stores that sell kitchen items, although it might be easier to just use the packaging to estimate the serving size. Once you start to get the feel for serving sizes, which should take only a day or two, you'll be able to approximate serving size by looking. We recommend measuring serving sizes once in a while, though, to make sure you are still accurate.

The next part of the Pyramid is vegetables, and you should have three to five servings of vegetables each day. A serving is one cup of leafy green vegetables, a half cup of other vegetables (cooked or chopped raw), or 6 ounces of vegetable juice. People usually say they'd rather eat fruits than vegetables, but in reality, Americans eat more vegetables. How can that be? One reason is that we eat a lot of vegetables as condiments (for example, lettuce, tomato, onion, and pickle on a hamburger).

Also, we tend to eat "camouflaged" vegetables, such as those found in a meatloaf or stew.

The Pyramid recommends two to three servings of fruits each day. A serving is one medium apple or banana, a half cup of canned or chopped fruit, or six ounces of fruit juice. You may have heard of the recommendation to eat "5 A Day" of vegetables and fruits. To come up with the number 5, health experts added the minimum number from vegetables (3) and the minimum number from fruits (2). It's important for everyone to eat foods rich in vitamins, minerals, and "phytonutrients" like lycopene and beta-carotene. As you feel ready to add some healthy habits to your smoke-free lifestyle, adding fruits and vegetables to your diet should be high on your list.

Milk, yogurt, and cheese make up the next part of the Pyramid, and we recommend two to three servings each day. A serving is one cup of milk or yogurt or two ounces of cheese. These foods are important because they provide calcium and vitamin D, which can help build strong bones. Researchers have found that in men, smoking negatively affects the production of bone cells. For women, smoking tends to lead to earlier menopause, which puts them at higher risk for osteoporosis. Some people don't like to drink milk or eat cheese because they find it gives them gas or diarrhea, and there are vegetarians who choose not to eat dairy products. Alternative sources of calcium include tofu, kale, broccoli, and greens (like mustard greens and turnip greens). Don't forget you can buy orange juice fortified with both calcium and vitamin D to help meet your nutrient needs. Nutrition is very personal. Feel free to tweak these recommendations, but just be sure you get enough calcium and vitamin D from foods (or supplements).

The last food group on the Pyramid is called "meat, poultry, dry beans, eggs, and nuts." These foods are good sources of protein so try to eat two to three servings each day. A serving is three ounces of meat, one egg, a half-cup of cooked beans, two

It's Not Just Any Old Carbohydrate

Over the last few years, there's been a lot in the news about high- versus low-carbohydrate diets. This discussion, however, has overlooked a very important difference in the kind of carbohydrates we eat. White bread, cakes, cookies, and sweets and desserts with refined carbohydrates can raise your blood sugar quickly and make you drowsy and hungry after about an hour. You are more likely to gain weight by eating this kind of carbohydrate. On the other hand, unrefined carbohydrates like whole wheat breads cause your blood sugar to rise more slowly so your body can process the sugar gradually without making you feel like you need a nap. As you choose breads, cereals, rice, and pasta, look for ones that have whole grains. Check out the list of ingredients and look for whole wheat flour or whole oats. These foods have more fiber, which is good for your heart. Another benefit of eating whole grains and other fiber-rich foods is that the fiber helps to fill you up while adding a low amount of calories. This way, you'll feel fuller between meals and may be less tempted to snack.

tablespoons of peanut butter, or one-third cup of nuts. As you can see, there are lots of ways to get protein in your diet. In fact, most Americans get much more protein than they really need.

The last part of the Pyramid is called "the tip." Sometimes, people try to put foods in here that don't really belong. (For example, french fries count as a vegetable, not as a "tip" food.) "Tip" foods include soft drinks, alcoholic beverages, candies, butter, and mayonnaise. Nutritionists recommend that these foods be eaten sparingly. As you quit smoking, it's likely that these tip foods will appeal to you, especially candies and chocolates. No foods are forbidden as you create your new nutrition lifestyle, but do keep in mind that these foods are high in calories and are not the best choices if you're trying to avoid gaining weight.

Key Foods for Ex-Smokers

In addition to your quitting smoking, there are some key changes in your diet that will help ward off some of the same diseases smoking can cause. Also, there are some things you can do to help your body recover from some of the negative effects of smoking. Here are some suggestions:

PHYTONUTRIENTS AND ANTIOXIDANTS

Of course, most of us know it's a good thing to eat vegetables. A specific reason for this is that many vegetables contain compounds, called **phytonutrients**. Some of these are also **antioxidants**, including vitamins E and C and beta-carotene (a plant pigment that we can convert to vitamin A in our bodies). Antioxidants can be found in vegetables and fruits such as broccoli, Brussels sprouts, cabbage, spinach, kale, turnip greens, carrots, yams, cantaloupe, butternut squash, and cauliflower. Tomatoes, watermelon, and red peppers contain lycopene, which is an antioxidant that can lower the risk of prostate cancer for men. Other phytonutrients are also found in garlic and onions and can stimulate enzymes that reduce the risk of stomach cancer, lower blood pressure, and strengthen the immune system.

The antioxidants and other phytonutrients can help your body fight some of the same diseases you are trying to avoid by quitting smoking. These include coronary heart disease and a number of kinds of cancers.

Research shows that many smokers don't eat many foods that are rich in antioxidants, and therefore, are especially at risk for illness. So it just makes sense to focus on eating these foods when you quit, sort of like protecting your investment in the health benefits of both quitting smoking and "eating your vegetables."

VITAMIN C

Free radicals are chemicals that can damage cells and shut down cell function. The free radicals in cigarette smoke cause your body to have less vitamin C than it should—even if you've been drinking lots of orange juice. Smokers expose themselves to incredibly high levels of free radicals. This means that folks quitting smoking may have to overcome a long history of doing this to their bodies. They need extra vitamin C in order to get their body's levels of this critical vitamin back up to normal. Some great sources of vitamin C include citrus fruits, strawberries, tomatoes, and potatoes.

Power Foods to Aid Quitting Smoking and Managing Your Weight

Many foods have across-the-board positive effects to help the body become healthy again after you quit smoking. These include foods that can help boost your immune system. Eating well can stave off infection, prevent disease, and keep you in optimum health, especially when you eat foods such as citrus fruits, garlic, yogurt, mushrooms, and many others that work to strengthen your immune system.

In the upcoming chapters, we'll build on what you've already learned about maintaining a balanced diet and adopting healthy eating habits with more detailed information about foods that can help you become healthier, fight cancer and other diseases, and control your weight after you quit smoking.

Let's get started!

Preparing to Quit:
The First 2–3 Weeks

3

"*I was really worried about my health so I decided to quit smoking. One day I went to dinner at a friend's house and he offered me a cigarette after dessert. I broke down and had one. Before I knew it, I was back to smoking a pack a day. More recently, I tried to quit, but this time I took it slowly and really planned for it. I told my friend that I wanted to stop smoking cigarettes so he wouldn't offer me one again. Wouldn't you know it, he wanted to quit too.*" (Peter, age 34)

Now that you have completed your introductory lesson to a healthy lifestyle, it's time to turn some of those ideas into practice. You can probably see where Peter went wrong: the most effective way to quit usually involves some planning, including getting support from your friends ahead of time.

As the case of Peter shows, just deciding to quit, no matter how determined you are, does not always mean you'll succeed. Statistics show that most initial decisions to quit smoking are usually followed by periods of relapse. But this does not have to happen to you. With a little planning, you can avoid some of the pitfalls. Think of it this way: quitting smoking is like building a house—its stability really depends on the foundation you lay. Physical activity, healthy eating, a nurturing support network, and a solid plan of action are your building blocks, not only for your success in quitting smoking but in developing a healthy lifestyle.

When preparing to quit smoking, two things should be kept in mind: first, quitting is not an event. It is a process. Whether you have tried to quit before or are doing so for the first time, quitting requires commitment on your part. Commitment does not mean rushing toward your goal, but rather, taking the time to figure out a plan you will be able to stick to in order to achieve your goal. That said, it's okay if you don't feel quite ready to quit at this point. We will help you prepare and build up to it.

Second, although time frames are important in managing your quitting process, they should not be too rigid. A "one size fits all" approach that is too hasty or strict carries a high potential for failure, which may only leave you frustrated. We want to help make this process as painless as possible. This means taking your time. Remember that doing it right means doing what's right for you. No two people are the same and plans to quit smoking should fit your everyday activities, not disrupt them.

In this chapter, we will prepare you for the weeks leading up to your Quit Day. Let's start by looking more closely at other parts of your life to see how we can get them to work in your favor. As Sun Tzu's *Art of War* says, "Every battle is won before it is actually fought." With some strategy and skill, the battle between you and your smoking habit can indeed be won!

How to Use the Upcoming Chapters in This Book

In this chapter, we focus on preparing you to stop smoking. We understand that not all people are ready to do the things they know they should do, and this is especially true for quitting smoking. In behavior change, it's often smarter to start where you are most likely to succeed or where you would most enjoy the challenge, rather than where you most need to make a change. A small success can actually be a big step, and can build your confidence and set the tone for future challenges.

Ask yourself the following questions: before you picked up this book, were you planning to quit within the next month? Have you made some actual quit attempts in the last 6 months and been able to not smoke for at least a day or so? If the answer to both of these is "no," you may want to think twice about trying to quit right away. If

> **COMMON REASONS WHY PEOPLE QUIT**
> - for my health
> - for the health of my family
> - (for pregnant women) to give my baby a healthy start
> - to set a good example for my family
> - for the health of people around me
> - to be in control of my body and my life
> - to look better
> - to save money
> - to feel better in general

you aren't quite sure yet about quitting, take it slow, and work through some of the exercises in this book to boost your motivation. We encourage you to photocopy the Action Items that appear in the upcoming chapters to use as worksheets. Remember, quitting smoking is the best thing you can do for your health, but at this point, you don't have to do everything at once. We want to get you thinking about your smoking habit and help you find ways to prepare to quit.

Preparing to Quit Smoking

Understanding Your Reasons for Quitting

"My three-year-old son used to cough all the time when I smoked. I felt bad about it and decided it was a good reason to quit. Every time I felt tempted to smoke, I took out his picture. There's no way I could have a cigarette after that!" (Michelle, age 45)

As you can imagine, Michelle's reason for quitting was a powerful force in keeping her smoke-free. Perhaps you have a similar reason for wanting to quit. On the lines below, make

---

QUITTING IS CRITICAL FOR PREGNANT WOMEN

When you smoke, you breathe in poisons that get into your blood and keep your baby from getting the food and oxygen he needs to grow. The sooner you quit, the sooner you can stop passing on all these poisons to your baby. Smokers are more likely to have a miscarriage; have the baby too soon; have trouble giving birth; have a baby that's stillborn or has a low birth weight; have a baby that dies soon after birth; and/or have a baby that gets sick frequently.

HOW SMOKE AFFECTS THE HEALTH OF NEARBY CHILDREN

Studies show that the health of babies and children is endangered when they inhale the smoke from other people's cigarettes, cigars, and pipes. In fact, children of parents who smoke are more likely to have chest colds, ear infections, bronchitis, and pneumonia than those whose parents are nonsmokers. Children who have asthma and who breathe secondhand smoke have more asthma attacks than those unexposed to secondhand smoke.

---

a list of your reasons for quitting. Try to think of as many as you can and why they are important to you. Take your time and make the list as detailed as possible. Some of the people we've worked with who have successfully quit have found it helpful to make copies of their lists and post them around their homes, offices—even the car. Other people have chosen to type out a list on a piece of paper the size of a business card and then laminate it and keep it in their purse or wallet. When the urge to smoke comes or you encounter some obstacles, having your list readily available can help remind you of why you are quitting in the first place and how important it is for you and the people in your life.

My Reasons for Quitting

Example:
I want to get pregnant and want to quit smoking before I do.

Example:
I know smoking is really bad for me and is making it difficult for me to exercise.

_____

_____

_____

_____

_____

_____

Remember, *quitting smoking is the most important thing you will do in the next year.* A year from now, you will feel wonderful if you have successfully quit smoking. This means that you've got to give quitting the attention that *the most important thing you will do all year* deserves. If you have to miss a couple of card games because too many of the other players smoke, or if you have to miss a party because there will be too many smokers around, so be it. Quitting—and your health and your future—deserve to be your top priorities.

Choosing a Quit Day

Now that you have identified your reasons for quitting, it's time to set a Quit Day. This is the date you will begin your smoke-free life. We'll go into the nuts and bolts of what will happen on the day itself in the next chapter, but rather than shrinking from setting a date, make it a day to remember! You could start it off by sleeping a little later than usual, taking a nice long walk, or taking a bubble bath—anything that makes you feel happy and relaxed. Think about whether you will want to be alone or with other people—and if with others, whom? Your Quit Day should be about 2 weeks from now—close enough that you can see it coming and far enough in the future that you can do some things to prepare for it.

When planning your Quit Day, try to avoid days that coincide with times you usually smoke. For example, if you tend to smoke at work, try quitting on a day off. If you smoke while socializing or going out on the town, quit on a weekday. The point is to free your day of associations that might tempt you to smoke. There's no reason to make it any harder than it already is. Another thing to consider in setting your Quit Day is its meaning to you. You may want to make it your birthday—or perhaps your spouse's or your grandchild's. Many people choose to make big changes or resolutions on New Year's Day, but you might want to think seriously about how you celebrate the new year and whether you'll have the energy or be in the best frame of mind to begin your plan for quitting.

At this point, we just want you to set a date that will feel like your own and put your goal clearly in sight. Once you decide on your Quit Day, write it in the space below, and mark it on all your calendars and datebooks both at home and at work.

My Quit Day: _____

Getting Encouragement and Cooperation from Family and Friends

Research shows that cooperation and encouragement from the folks around you are vital to making any change in your life. Support can be found in your family, but not only there. Co-workers, friends, members of your social club, or church are all people you can recruit to be on your support team. When it comes to motivation and how others can help, it is clearly up to you. Some may want a celebration, others a simple pat on the back, and still others singing telegrams. Examine what will work for you and then let the significant people in your life know about it. Tell them how important quitting is to you and how you are counting on their help.

Nobody can quit for you, but they surely can cooperate with you. Ask your friends who smoke not to offer you a cigarette and, at least in those most challenging times, not to smoke around you. You can even put this in writing in the form of a "contract" or provide them with information and resource materials, such as the American Lung Association's brochure on "How to Help a Friend Quit Smoking." You may

ACTION ITEM

Make a list of friends, co-workers, and others in your daily life. Let them know you are trying to quit smoking and ask for their support. Among the people on that list, try to identify one or two coaches. Sit down one-on-one and make a plan for how they can help you. Try to build a lot of contact into your plan, especially on your Quit Day and the couple of weeks after. You may also want to call a family meeting to tell your family members.

FRIENDS AND FAMILY WHO CAN HELP ME TO QUIT SMOKING

Name	What I Am Going to Ask Them to Do	Contacted yet?
Example: My spouse	Be there to support me when I am frustrated and craving a cigarette	Yes
Example: My co-worker	Take a walk with me after lunch instead of having a cigarette break	Yes

also want to ask a close friend or two to act as your accountability partner or quitting "coach." Having a coach to work with you can get you through difficult times. You could ask your coach to call and check in with you. A few words of encouragement could be what you need if you start to feel discouraged. A phone call can also help you fight a craving. After a few minutes on the phone, the urge to smoke is likely to pass.

Key Point: Nobody can read another's mind—unless you say what you want, your friends and family may do the wrong thing when trying to be helpful. They may ask you how quitting smoking is going when you don't want to talk about it or tell you to "look on the bright side" when all you want is to talk about how much you miss cigarettes. Tell them how you need them to help.

Remember that the battle against smoking is harder to win when it's fought alone!

Planning Ahead: Laying the Groundwork for a Healthy, Smoke-Free Life

Quitting smoking, physical activity, and healthy eating are the foundation for a healthy lifestyle. By adding some physical activity to your day and making very basic, simple changes in your eating habits, you can start to lay the groundwork for a healthy, smoke-free life. If you haven't been active, try doing 10 minutes of floor exercises each morning or evening. This may include doing some basic stretches such as sitting with your legs extended in front of you (or in a V-shape) and reaching for the tips of your toes, doing arm circles while sitting or standing, and rotating your shoulders, head, and ankles. Lunges are a good way to loosen up the muscles in your legs.

Walk It Off!

Another way to delay the urge to smoke is to walk it off. Walks can be particularly helpful because they are a fantastic distraction and don't require any planning. You can just get up and go when you start to feel the urge to smoke. They can also help you start to build your stamina for adding more physical activity to your daily routine when you are ready, and can have a positive effect on your efforts to manage your weight. In the next chapter, we'll give you more detailed advice on how to get more physically active, but for now decide to take a 2-, 5- or 10-minute walk each time you feel a craving to take your mind off cigarettes and onto the healthy new you.

If you already lead an active lifestyle, make a point of doing some kind of physical activity, such as playing tennis, riding a bike, going for a long walk—at least a few times during the next week.

You can also start to make a difference by making some minor change in your eating habits. Try to find just one or two specific ways you would enjoy (or hardly mind) improving your diet, such as substituting fruit for one sweet dessert each day, or switching from mayonnaise to mustard on your sandwich. Many salad dressings have low-calorie alternatives, or you can take some of the advice from chapter two, and try adding an extra vegetable to your daily eating routine. You might also choose to focus on your beverage intake by switching from whole milk to 1% or fat-free milk, or replacing your regular soda with a low-calorie version, flavored water, or sugar-free iced tea. The idea for now is just to make a small change or two. Baby steps can help you to quit smoking, and also help in managing your weight.

Where, When and Why You Smoke

Knowing the where, when, and why of your smoking habit can help you plan ahead for the times when a cigarette is most tempting. Here is where you begin to track your smoking habits and identify parts of the day when you are most likely to smoke. This tracking method has been used for over a quarter century in American Lung Association programs and has proven to be an integral part of helping thousands of people better understand their smoking habit and learn how to break it.

The Secret of Fighting Temptations

There are two keys to prevent being undone by temptations after you quit. The first is to anticipate temptation. If you wait for one to strike before coming up with a plan to fight it, then you may be too late. With the records you've kept here and some reflection, you can anticipate and be prepared for those times when you're most likely to be tempted to smoke. The second key to avoid giving in to a temptation is to have a specific plan for how you will deal with it. "I'll just have to be very careful when that happens" is not a specific plan. Figure out exactly what you will do if and when the temptation surfaces.

Especially in the first few weeks after quitting, one way of dealing with temptations is to avoid them. If everybody on your bowling team smokes, you may need to miss a few weeks of bowling. If your normal time to take a break at work is with several smokers, speak to your boss and your colleagues about switching your break. If driving to work in the car really brings on cravings, try to take the bus or the train. Be creative when coming up with ways to avoid succumbing to your temptations and keep in mind that what works best for another person may not work for you.

ACTION ITEM

Track your smoking habit for three or four days. Make photocopies of the chart on the next page for each day. On Day One, put a copy of the chart in your wallet or cigarette pack and carry it around with you wherever you go. Use a rubber band to attach the list to your pack if needed. Do this for three or four days, preferably over a time period that includes a weekday and a day during the weekend.

For each cigarette you have on a given day, record the time and place you had it. Then consider how badly you felt you needed it. Enter one exclamation mark (!) if you could take it or leave it, two (!!) for when you wanted to smoke but were not overcome by the desire, and three (!!!) if you were absolutely dying for a cigarette.

In the column titled "How Did I Feel?" make some notes on how you were feeling at the time. Maybe you felt relaxed or were having a good time with friends, or perhaps you were stressed out at work and had a cigarette to calm your nerves. Think about your mood and state of mind as you track your smoking habit, and write it down in the space provided.

After you've tracked your smoking habits for three or four days, pull out your sheets and look them over.

Now look at the column titled "How Much Did I Need It?" In the table below, write down the time, place, and how you felt when you had the strongest urge to smoke.

MY MOST IMPORTANT CIGARETTES

Cigarette #1	Cigarette #2	Cigarette #3
Time	Time	Time
Place	Place	Place
How I Felt	How I Felt	How I Felt

Date:

Cig #	Time of Day	Place	How Much Did I Need It? (! - !! - !!!)	How Did I Feel?
1				
2				
3				
4				
5				
6				
7				
8				
9				
10				
11				
12				
13				
14				
15				
16				
17				
18				
19				
20				

Note: *If some of these needs seem strong or overwhelming, you may want to think again about using nicotine gum or nicotine patches or talking to your doctor about prescription drugs that may be helpful to you.*

Another way of coping with temptations is to make specific plans so that wherever you are, you'll have something to do instead of smoking. Look at the time, place, and how you were feeling during your three most important cigarettes. Start to think about how you can replace smoking with physical activity or a healthy snack from the list on pages 81–83 in chapter four. Here are some ideas:

Things to Do Instead of Smoking

Now take a look at the table where you indicated your most important cigarettes. If you found that your urges were strongest when you were feeling relaxed or enjoying yourself, try to find some alternatives to smoking in the table below:

General	Physical Activity	Healthy Eating
Do a puzzle	Take a brisk walk	Prepare a healthy dessert for your family
See a movie	Go dancing	Have a non-alcoholic drink, like a piña colada with pineapple juice and a banana
Go shopping	Go to the park and play with the kids	Have a healthy snack, such as a fruit salad (see pages 81–83 for more suggestions)

If you tended to need a cigarette more when you were bored or needed something to do, then try the following instead:

General	Physical Activity	Healthy Eating
Call a friend	Work on a home improvement project	Shop for some fresh fruits and prepare a fruit salad snack
Read a book	Take a swim or bike ride	Drink some water or iced tea
Start a diary or put old photos in an album	Call a friend for a game of racquetball or a walk	Make a smoothie (see recipe on page 82)

If you found that your most critical cigarettes were when you were stressed, upset, or angry, then the following suggestions might help you get through it:

General	Physical Activity	Healthy Eating
Call a supportive friend	Put on an exercise video and do Tae Bo, kickboxing or whatever will help work out your frustration	Eat a healthy snack, perhaps something chewy or crunchy such as a low-calorie fig bar, raisins, or graham crackers
Put on your earphones and listen to your favorite music, as loud as you want	Do the relaxation exercise on page 72	Make some hot herbal tea and try to relax
Squeeze a ball or snap a rubber band to release tension	Jump rope, shoot baskets, or hit some golf balls	Chop some fresh veggies for a dinner salad or in-between snack

Relaxation Exercise

STEP 1: Think about something that makes you feel good.

STEP 2: Relax your shoulders. Close your mouth. Inhale slowly and as deeply as you can. Keep your shoulders relaxed.

STEP 3: Hold your breath while you count to four.

STEP 4: Exhale slowly, letting out all the air from your lungs.

STEP 5: Slowly repeat these steps five times.

Rewards

Even though quitting can be tough, it doesn't have to be painful. Rewards can get you through the hard times and help reinforce your decision to quit. And they don't have to be too extravagant or cost too much. They just have to be things that make you feel good. Use your rewards to celebrate milestones in your quitting process, such as getting past a roadblock or making it through your Quit Day. Make a list of things you can reward yourself with. Make sure to keep this list handy, and reward yourself for milestones in quitting, but also for increasing physical activity and making healthy eating choices.

The following are some rewards you might enjoy:

- Sleep late
- Get some fresh flowers for your home
- Take a bubble bath
- Schedule a massage
- Buy a new CD or magazine
- Have a day of beauty at your salon
- Buy running shoes or exercise equipment

- Call a faraway friend or family member for a long chat
- Go to a show or sporting event
- Go shopping
- Spend extra time on a favorite hobby
- Go to a movie or rent one of your favorites
- Eat a special (healthy) meal
- Spend some time with good friends
- Take pictures or look through old photo albums
- Eat dinner at a new restaurant in town
- Read a book
- Go for a relaxing walk
- Go to a museum
- Buy some new tools

Overcoming Roadblocks

Even in the best circumstances, there are obstacles to overcome when quitting smoking. Roadblocks are very common. Everyone has them. The trick is to not let them discourage you from quitting and staying smoke-free for good. You can plan ways to get past them. The Action Item in this section will help you do just that.

When thinking about your personal roadblocks to quitting, remember that there are different kinds. Some are mental and have to do with how you view your smoking habit. Others have to do with your social life and how much support you'll have when you quit. Still others are related to what you think might happen if you quit, such as gaining weight or being irritable.

Here are examples of some common roadblocks people face when trying to quit.

- *I am worried about gaining weight.*
  Weight gain can be a real problem. But there are many ways you can avoid or minimize that gain with healthy eating habits and by making physical activity a bigger part of your

life. In chapter seven, we will give you more details on how to manage your weight after you quit smoking.

♦ *Smoking is part of my routine.*
Routines are not set in stone. Experimenting even slightly with your daily routines by adding new, healthier activities such as walking, reading a book, or trying a new hobby, will take you out of your smoking rut and other unhealthy activities.

♦ *My friends all smoke and it will be too hard to stop around them.*
Spending time with friends who smoke can make it hard for you to quit. The same goes for members of your family. Try getting their support ahead of time. Tell them how important it is for you to quit and how they can help. They will be impressed by your resolve and may even want to join you. Refer back to page 63 on "Getting Encouragement and Cooperation from Family and Friends."

♦ *When I don't smoke, I feel fidgety, like I need to do something with my hands.*
Try to focus your attention on other things. You can keep your hands busy by cooking, gardening, sewing, writing a letter, or munching on a carrot or celery stick. You may also want to try the relaxation exercise on page 72—it can do wonders for calming you and helping you regain your sense of well-being.

♦ *I get nervous and irritable without smoking.*
Nervousness and irritability can be overcome. Physical activity can improve your mood and leave you with an overall sense of well-being. Use the relaxation exercise to get you through the tense moments and cravings. You may also find it helpful to line up some substitutes for when you are going to miss smoking the most; try some of the sug-

gestions on page 70 in this chapter under the heading "Things to Do Instead of Smoking."

+ *Smoking gives me extra energy and keeps me going.*
There are other things you can do to boost your energy level. Physical activity is a great way to get re-energized and can build your stamina over time. A balanced diet full of vitamins and nutrients can also keep you at a good energy level. Chapter five will give you more details on how to build and maintain your energy level while trying to kick the habit over the long run.

+ *There are a lot of problems in life.*
Many smokers have other stressors in their lives besides quitting smoking. If you are going through or recovering from a major loss or problem, this may not be the best time to quit. But keep this book around and come back to it when you feel ready. And you might still want to adopt some of the physical activity and healthy diet recommendations in this book so you can feel you are being good to yourself. Changes in these areas can pave the way to eventually quitting smoking.

There is no "right time" to quit smoking. Quitting is tough, but as we've said, 49 percent of all smokers have done it and you can too. Also, quitting can make you feel more positive. You may find that some of the tools you use to quit smoking can help you tackle other problems.

+ *Without cigarettes, I will feel lost.*
There are so many good things in life that can fill the gaps once you've left smoking behind. You can make it easier to quit by filling your time with other things such as calling a friend, seeing a movie, going to a museum, spending more time with your family, or exercising.

ACTION ITEM

In the space below, list all the barriers that you think stand in the way of quitting smoking. Once you have identified your road-blocks, think about how to handle them. In the second column, next to each roadblock, list some ways of getting past them. Draw from the above examples if they apply to you.

Roadblock	How to Get Past It
1. Example: Smoking is part of my routine.	I will take a 2-minute walk each time I want to smoke.
2. Example: When I feel nervous or angry, smoking calms me.	Each time I get upset I will do the relaxation exercises in this chapter to calm myself.
3.	
4.	
5.	
6.	

How did you do? If you had a long list of roadblocks or couldn't think of how to get around them right away, don't be frustrated. You can always go back and fill in the blanks later on. In fact, in the upcoming chapters, you'll learn several strategies and handy tips using physical activity and healthy eating to overcome some of your roadblocks over time. If you do, be sure to add them to your list.

Remember, roadblocks are only temporary. They might slow you down a bit, but getting past them can really feel great, especially when you get to those rewards. By completing the exercises in this chapter, you've laid a strong foundation for quitting smoking. In the next chapter, we'll focus specifically on your Quit Day—the first day of your smoke-free life.

Preparing for and Getting Through Your Quit Day

4

"I remember my Quit Day because it was such a great day! I decided to do it on a Saturday because weekends are less stressful for me. My family wanted to support me so we spent the day together, having a nice breakfast and later going to the museum. I also took a walk with my neighbor. She wanted to be part of the day. She even called later to check in and make sure I was okay." (Ellen, age 50)

My Quit Day is: _____

So you've just about made it to the big day—the first day of your smoke-free life. Now you can use all the great prep work you did in the first three chapters to actually quit. Remember, by quitting you are adding years to your life and making sure they're quality years by improving your eating habits and increasing your level of physical activity. It's tough, but it could be one of your greatest achievements ever.

In chapters one through three, you laid the foundation for quitting smoking. You learned about the importance of good nutrition and physical activity, and how both can help you quit and manage your weight. In this chapter, we'll take you step-by-step through the process of making it work. This means preparing your home and work environments and making a solid plan for what you'll do on your Quit Day. It also includes creating strategies for combating cravings and coping with some of the more difficult feelings you may experience on your Quit Day and the weeks following. We'll focus very specifically on combating those urges to eat unhealthy foods in place of smoking, since these urges tend to be at their worst during the first two weeks. We'll show you how to use healthy foods, snacks, and beverages to fight off the urge to binge or snack on foods that are high in fat and sugars, and provide you with a list of healthier alternatives that will help you to quit smoking and avoid gaining weight in the process.

Preparing Your Home and Work Environment for Your Quit Day

Buy Your Quit-Smoking Aids

If you smoke more than a pack a day, you may especially want to consider using nicotine gum or patches, or discuss other prescription medications with your doctor. Reread the section on "Smoking and Addiction" in chapter two (page 30) and consult your doctor to learn more about your options. If you plan to use a quit aid such as nicotine gum or patches, you can find them in most drug stores or large supermarkets with drug departments. Be sure to carefully follow the directions on the packaging, and if you plan to use nicotine gum, make sure to avoid eating and drinking for at least 15 minutes before chewing it and an additional 15 minutes while chewing it to prevent reduced absorption of the nicotine. Especially avoid drinking acidic beverages, such as coffee or soft drinks that can interfere with the efficacy of the gum. If you are using Zyban® (available only by prescription), remember to follow the instructions, paying special attention to timing (you must start using it far enough in advance of your Quit Day so that it is working for you by the time you need it).

Get Rid of Your Cigarettes

Before your Quit Day, throw away all of the cigarettes in your home or anywhere else you may have a stash: in the pocket of your coat, in the car, or in the office. Do the same with lighters, ashtrays, and matches. Make it impossible to get a cigarette without going to a lot of trouble.

Stock up on Healthy Snacks

Eating healthy snacks is a great way to get you through your Quit Day and satisfy the craving to smoke. Place a bowl of fruit on the kitchen table and stock your cupboard with some low-calorie, easy-to-grab foods. Having healthy snacks around the house and your workspace can help when you need something to satisfy your urge to smoke. Below are some suggestions for healthy snack foods to stock up on before your Quit Day:

Beverages:

- Low-calorie beverages, such as sugar-free iced tea, sodas, and flavored waters.

Produce:

- Your favorite (raw) vegetables. Carrots, celery, cauliflower, and peppers are great snacks; try them with low-fat dressing or cottage cheese.

- Fruits: apples to eat on your way to work or for baking with cinnamon and a teaspoon of sugar. Buy ingredients for fruit salad or delicious smoothies, using peaches, plums, pineapple (fresh or canned), pears, cantaloupe, blueberries, raspberries, or strawberries. Don't forget to look in the frozen food aisle at the store because you'll be able to find an assortment of frozen fruits that are great to eat cold.

SMOOTHIES

Smoothies are a great breakfast choice and can be a terrific snack in the middle of the day. You can fulfill your fruit servings and satisfy your hunger and cravings for sweets. Simply take your favorite fruits and blend them with ice, milk, or with low- or non-fat frozen yogurt. You can even use orange or pineapple juices as a fat-free alternative to milk or yogurt. The following are some ideas for fruit combinations you might enjoy:

- Peach, pineapple, and mango
- Carrot, banana, orange, and yogurt
- Mixed berries and pineapple
- Strawberry, banana, and apple
- Pineapple, raspberry, and papaya

Non-Perishables:

- The snack and cereal aisles can offer some sweet and crunchy alternatives such as low-calorie fruit bars and fig bars, oven-baked chips and pretzels, air-popped or low-fat popcorn. Also try wheat or graham crackers, rice cakes, ready-to-eat cereal (to munch on, without milk), or shredded wheat. Buy sugarless gum or candy to keep around the office or in your purse, briefcase, or backpack.

Frozen Foods:

♦ Frozen fruit bars, sugar-free popsicles, and low- or non-fat frozen yogurt are great desserts or in-between meal treats.

Dairy:

♦ Buy 1% or skim milk (mix with cocoa for sweetness if you like) and low-fat cheese sticks (string cheese).

DON'T BE TOO HARD ON YOURSELF

While eating fruits, carrot sticks, or other healthy foods is an excellent replacement for smoking, sometimes a piece of celery just doesn't satisfy and it's that piece of chocolate that you really crave. If a piece of chocolate will keep you from reaching for a cigarette, then so be it. Just be sure that if you are going to eat some of the more fattening or high-calorie foods, you do so in moderation. You don't have to deny yourself food, but keep in mind that the foods you're craving may be high in calories. Try eating an apple or a celery stick to satisfy most of your cravings, and reserve a piece of chocolate for the really tough craving. If you tend to snack on chips, replace them with baked chips or pretzels.

ACTION ITEM

HEALTHY SNACKING

Make a list of the snacks that you especially like and some healthier replacements for them. You can use this list for when you go shopping and stock up on healthy snacks, and for your Quit Day and afterwards—any time you find yourself craving a cigarette.

Snacks I Enjoy	Healthier Alternatives
Example: potato chips	Pretzels, rice cakes, air-popped popcorn
Example: chocolate ice cream	Frozen yogurt, low-fat chocolate milk

Planning Your Quit Day

Your Quit Day is a milestone in your life. It should be a special day—a day on which you treat yourself like royalty. On your Quit Day, be sure to do something you really enjoy, such as treating yourself to a dinner out, cooking a special meal, spending extra time on a hobby—anything that will keep your mind off smoking and make you feel relaxed and in a good mood.

ACTION ITEM

STOCK UP ON REWARDS

Quit Day is the most important day to have your rewards in place. Give yourself some tangible reasons not to smoke on this important day. Refer back to the list of rewards you made in chapter three and in the space below, list four or five of them that you will use specifically on your Quit Day.

1. _____

2. _____

3. _____

4. _____

5. _____

After you select some rewards, be sure to stock up on any last minute items you may need, such as a new book, bubble bath, or the video you've wanted to rent.

Now you should focus on what you will do on your Quit Day. Instead of being worried or nervous that you won't be able to do it, think about how you can fill the time with fun activities or some rest and relaxation. The following are some examples of how successful ex-smokers spent their Quit Day. Maybe you can take a few ideas for planning your day.

+ *"I went to the movies. You can't smoke there."*

+ *"I went to a day spa and got a massage and a manicure. I felt relaxed and ready to take on the world!"*

◆ *"I did some fixing up around the house. I had wanted to do it for a while. It kept my hands busy and my mind off smoking."*

◆ *"I went shopping and bought some new shoes. I figured I deserved it since I had been working so hard at quitting smoking."*

◆ *"I cooked a healthy meal with my family."*

◆ *"I worked. No one smokes there and it kept me busy. My co-workers were coming by my desk all day long and congratulating me. They were really supportive."*

What will you do on Quit Day? Use the chart below to schedule your first smoke-free day. Fill in the first three columns with where you will be at each time of the day, what you plan to do, and how you will reward yourself for getting through that part of the day without having a cigarette. Take a look at some of the suggestions under each of the time frames in the row titled "How Physical Activity and Healthy Eating Can Help" to see how you can use what you have learned so far to help get you through the day. The following example can help:

Time and Place	General Activities	Rewards
Morning 7:00 am – 11:00 am		
Saturday morning at home with the family.	Eat a healthy breakfast.	Sleep late and take a long bubble bath before or after breakfast.
Monday morning at work.	Have a healthy breakfast. Organize my day so that I can do some of the more simple tasks and save the tougher ones for the next day.	Step outside for a moment at some point during the morning, take a leisurely walk, and if possible, buy some fresh flowers for my desk.

Quit Day Planner

My Quit Day: _____

Time and Place	General Activities	Rewards
Morning Time 7:00 – 11:00 am		

How Physical Activity and Healthy Eating Can Help

- Have a healthy breakfast: prepare a fruit salad the night before. Eat some oatmeal topped off with cinnamon or honey. Or try making a fruit smoothie using the directions on page 82 of this chapter.
- Keep some of the healthy snacks listed on pages 81–83 on hand (at home or office), such as a fruit salad, dried fruit (like raisins), and some chewing gum for the times when you crave a cigarette.
- If you feel yourself reaching for a cigarette while at work, take a brisk walk and let the urge pass.
- If you decide to quit over a weekend, try to plan a physical activity, such as a trip to the park or a day at the beach for a nice, mid-morning swim. In the winter months, you might choose to go skating with the kids or some friends.

Afternoon 11:00 – 3:00 pm		

How Physical Activity and Healthy Eating Can Help

- Have a healthy lunch: if you are not at home, make sure to pack a lunch, and if you are at home, try to take your time and make something you will enjoy. Or, keep your hands busy by making a healthy dessert for after dinner. (Chapter nine is full of great lunch ideas and recipes.)

Continued on next page

Continued from previous page

- At work, have some herbal tea during your coffee break instead of going outside for a smoke.
- When you crave a cigarette at work, try walking up stairs to release nervous energy.
- If you are at home, go for a leisurely bike ride.

Evening *3:00 – 7:00 pm*		

HOW PHYSICAL ACTIVITY AND HEALTHY EATING CAN HELP

- Cook one of the dinner recipes in chapter nine with your family or invite some friends over to cook with you.
- If you decide to quit on a work day, try starting a new after-work dance or low-impact aerobics class.
- Take an evening swim at the community pool.

Nighttime *7:00 – 11:00 pm*		

HOW PHYSICAL ACTIVITY AND HEALTHY EATING CAN HELP

- If you get the urge to have a late snack, try some fruit, or skim or 1% milk with cocoa.
- Do some floor exercises in front of the TV such as sit-ups, stretches, leg lifts, and arm circles.
- Put on an exercise video and follow along for a half hour or so.

Coping with Nicotine Withdrawal over the Next Two to Three Weeks

In the next two to three weeks without cigarettes, you may feel more sleepy or lightheaded, or overly excited and irritable. You may have cravings for sweet or salty foods at times when you used to smoke. These are signs that the nicotine is leaving your body. Your body got used to the nicotine and now that you have taken it away, it's asking you for more.

Remember that many of these physical symptoms will go away within the first couple of weeks. After the first week, much of the nicotine will have left your system and with it your body's reaction to the immediate loss of a chemical that it had become used to. After that, you will still have cravings and other reactions, but these cravings will be based on the psychological associations you have developed, such as not being able to enjoy your morning coffee without a cigarette. But these associations will lessen over time.

The best thing you can do at this stage is to know what to look for and to plan how you'll cope when cravings happen and symptoms occur. The better you can anticipate times when you are going to be tempted to smoke and the more you have specific plans for managing them, the more easily you will negotiate the next few weeks. Even if a temptation sneaks up on you and catches you unaware, it's still good to have thought through the specific things you can do to get past it without smoking.

You've already learned how to cope with nicotine cravings by using healthy snacks and delaying the urge to smoke. The following are suggestions for how to handle some of the other sensations you may experience as the nicotine leaves your body. These were developed from our own work with patients and decades of American Lung Association programs that have helped thousands of people quit and stay smoke-free.

- **Fatigue, Feeling Extra Tired**

  For many people, nicotine acts as a stimulant. Now that you have quit, your body is going back to normal. If you feel extra tired or sluggish, try to reserve some extra time for sleeping. Let yourself take naps and don't push yourself too hard. Remember, you can't smoke when you are asleep. On the other hand, another way to overcome feelings of fatigue is to exercise. Chapter five is full of suggestions.

- **Dizziness, Headaches**

  If you feel dizzy, make sure to move around a little more slowly and carefully and be extra cautious. Unless you and your doctor have decided you shouldn't use them, you can try over-the-counter, nonprescription pain medicines like aspirin or ibuprofen to get rid of a headache. You might try cold compresses or taking a warm bath or hot shower when you feel a headache coming on. You can also drink more water and reduce your intake of caffeine. Try cutting down or replacing your morning coffee with herbal tea, or start making your coffee half decaffeinated.

- **Coughing, Sore Throat, Nasal Drip**

  It may seem strange to be coughing more after you quit, but there's a good reason for it. Healthy lungs are equipped with cells that help to clean out dust and other substances so that you can breathe. In smokers' lungs, these cells don't always work the way they are supposed to, which is why smokers tend to be more prone to infection. Within the first couple of weeks after your Quit Day, your lungs start to clear away the stuff built up in them from your smoking. This is a sign that they are starting to heal. There is no quick fix for lung repair, but cough drops and hard candy can help offset coughing fits, and, again, be sure to drink plenty of water.

◆ Difficulty Concentrating

For many people, the nicotine in cigarettes helps make them feel more alert. Having difficulty concentrating is yet another sign of your body going back to normal and healing itself. You may be distracted by other symptoms you are experiencing—feeling extra tired or anxious can throw off your thought processes. Try some physical activity when you are feeling distracted. If you are at your desk and can't seem to focus on your work, get up and take a short walk. A 5-minute walk might clear your head and help you focus. Stretching and relaxation exercises can also calm you down. You might also try to lessen your workload for the next couple of weeks and avoid additional stress.

◆ Stress, Irritability, Nervousness, Difficulty Sleeping

Stress and irritability are common symptoms of quitting smoking. If you have difficulty sleeping over the next couple of weeks, this is likely the reason. Your body is going through some serious changes and it is understandable that you will be stressed. Give yourself a break and don't expect too much. Also, ask your friends and family to understand if you are a little short-tempered—this is where your social supports can really help. Drink plenty of water to flush out the nicotine, and avoid drinks with caffeine in them, such as coffee or colas. You can replace the colas you usually drink with ones that are decaffeinated or with flavored seltzer water. Walks, hot baths, taking regular stretch breaks during the day, and doing the relaxation exercise from chapter three on page 72 can help calm you down, and physical activity is great for taking off the edge. Expend some of that nervous energy with some physical activity—go for a bike ride or leisurely swim, wash the car, or do some housework or gardening.

◆ Constipation, Stomach Gas, Stomach Pain

You can combat these symptoms by eating more fruits, vegetables, and whole grains. These foods can help to flush out your system. Try to drink 8–10 glasses of water per day. Physical activity can also help keep you regular. When you exercise on a regular basis, you decrease the amount of time that food hangs around in your body. Having the food move through your body faster results in less likelihood of constipation.

How was your first day as an ex-smoker? Remember, by making it through just one day without smoking, you have:

◆ put less strain on your heart and lowered your chance of having a heart attack;

◆ increased the amount of oxygen in your blood and the amount of oxygen going to your muscles when you exercise;

◆ shown yourself that you can actually do it.

Reward yourself for a job well done. It just gets easier from here!

Staying Smoke-free: Managing Your Weight Through Physical Activity

5

"I tried quitting smoking several times, but kept going back to it because I gained weight. I tried dieting and aerobics, but got frustrated and all I wanted to do was smoke. I didn't lose a pound. I decided to take a 2- or 5-minute walk each time I had the urge to smoke, and after a while, I had enough stamina to step up the pace to a jog. Now, I jog regularly. I don't even have the urge to smoke anymore, and I even started losing a little weight." (Angela, age 30)

It's official: you made it through your Quit Day. Quitting smoking is not an easy thing to do and taking those first steps can be trying. But you did it. And for that you should be very proud. If you haven't already done so, reward yourself. Now that you have begun your new, smoke-free life, let's work on keeping it that way by working on other aspects of your health, namely, physical activity.

Physical activity is one of the best ways to work on both your health and your appearance. There are countless benefits to being active, including the fact that it can help you stay smoke-free and manage your weight. Like Angela, many people

ACTION ITEM

GETTING ENCOURAGEMENT FROM FAMILY AND FRIENDS

As you start to become more active, remember that there are many activities that are simply more fun to do with other people—like going to the park, walking around the block, or going out dancing.

Make a list of friends, co-workers, and other people in your daily life. You might want to refer to the list of people you put together in chapter three (on page 64) to help you quit smoking. After you make the list, tell them that you are trying to quit smoking and get more active. Ask for support and encouragement in your decision, and ask if they would like to start doing some regular physical activity with you. You may need to work through the next couple of sections of this chapter before you can decide which activities are right for you. But you can start to get the support of your friends and family and see who's interested in joining you. Perhaps you can brainstorm together the kind of activities you would like to do. The sidebar on page 104 can help you get started.

get caught in the cycle of quitting, gaining weight, and going back to smoking because of the weight they gain. But you can use physical activity to avoid or at least minimize that weight gain, while working on kicking your smoking habit for good.

In this chapter we will focus more closely on physical activity and how it can help you if you are struggling to quit smoking or have already quit and are trying to stay smoke-free. One of the ways that physical activity helps is by giving you something to do instead of smoking. When some people quit, they feel that something important has been taken away from them. One of the best ways to get over that feeling of loss is to fill those empty spaces with new habits and activities. Physical activity is a great alternative because it can be fun and it's incompatible with smoking—you simply can't smoke when you are walking, jogging, swimming, playing tennis, gardening, or housecleaning. Physical activity can help get you through some difficult times, such as when you are really craving a cigarette, feeling irritable and/or stressed out.

Research has shown that regular, vigorous physical activity can help people to stay off cigarettes and manage their weight. We also know that even moderate-intensity activity can help to manage your weight and is likely to help you stay smoke-free. Now this doesn't mean that you have to immediately start on a vigorous exercise program. Increasing your level of physical activity can be tough, especially if it's been a while since you've been active. Don't feel bad if you need to start out slowly; most people do. Or, if you are moving forward but need to take a couple of steps back, don't be too concerned—this is very common. The important thing is that you build up to a regular exercise routine that fits your lifestyle.

Keep in mind that becoming more active does not have to be painful. There are obstacles, but they can be overcome by planning ahead of time. We will help you find simple ways to fit physical activity into your life that don't require too much time or money. You can start by stepping up the things you already do—such as taking an extra lap around the mall when you go shopping or parking a little farther away from the grocery store and walking the extra distance. This can help you build up to a more vigorous level when you are ready.

Identifying Your Current Level of Activity

Let's consider the amount of physical activity you are prepared to do and how often you can do it. In order to find out what you are ready for, you first need to know what you are already doing. Here, we will take you through a time study of your daily routines with an eye on finding out how active you are right now and where you might be able to fit in more physical activity.

ACTION ITEM

PERSONAL TIME STUDY OF PHYSICAL ACTIVITY
Make photocopies of the worksheet on the opposite page for each of the three days you will do your time study. Pick a mixture of weekend and weekdays. Starting in the morning, use the form throughout the day to list your daily activities. Make a note of every time you tended to smoke or still feel a strong craving to do so. Next to each activity, indicate whether you were physically active or not. Try to fill in the amount of time for each item.

Time Slot	Tasks/Activities/ Smoking?	Physically Active?
7:00 – 9:00 am	Having morning coffee (usually have a cigarette with the coffee)	No
1:00 – 3:00 pm	Sitting at my desk at work (usually take a smoke break at this time)	Yes, took a 10-minute walk.

Adapted from B.H. Marcus & L.H. Forsyth, 2003, *Motivating people to be physically active* (Champaign, IL: Human Kinetics), 103.

Personal Time Study of Physical Activity

Date:	Day of Week:	
Time Slot	**Tasks/Activities/ Smoking?**	**Physically Active?**
7:00 – 9:00 am		
9:00 – 11:00 am		
11:00 – 1:00 pm		
1:00 – 3:00 pm		
3:00 – 5:00 pm		
5:00 – 7:00 pm		
7:00 – 9:00 pm		
9:00 – 11:00 pm		
11:00 – 1:00 am		
1:00 – 3:00 am		
3:00 – 5:00 am		
5:00 – 7:00 am		

When doing your time study, try to think about the times of day you tended to smoke or when you felt (or still feel) a strong craving for a cigarette. You might want to refer back to the work you did in chapter three, especially in the section where you identified your "Most Important Cigarettes." Maybe you tended to smoke most when you were bored or inactive, and now that you've quit, you feel as if you need something to do. Our goal is to keep you from going back to smoking by filling the time with activity. In the time study you'll be looking more closely at your daily routines to see how physical activity can replace smoking and, more generally, how it can become a bigger part of your everyday life.

Overcoming Roadblocks to Physical Activity

Now that you have completed your personal time study, let's think about what might prevent you from becoming more active. All of us have personal barriers that may prevent us from being as physically active as we would like to be. Rest assured, there are ways to get past these barriers. The first thing to do is to identify some of the barriers ahead of time. Then you can figure out how to get past them when they become a problem.

Here is a list of common excuses people use to get out of making physical activity a part of their lives:

◆ *"I don't have the time."*
  Time is one of the main things people identify as a roadblock to physical activity. You may feel that your day is already too full, and fitting in physical activity is impossible or would be a major challenge. Try some of the chair

ACTION ITEM

Make a list of your roadblocks to physical activity. On the first line write down something that you think gets in your way of being more active. On the line underneath, write down a creative solution to getting past it. Do this for each roadblock you identify, and make sure to add to this list if you encounter any new ones down the line.

PHYSICAL ACTIVITY: OVERCOMING ROADBLOCKS

Roadblock: *Example:* No time to exercise after work.

How to Get Past it: Take a 10-minute walk at lunch each day and take a longer walk each weekend day.

Roadblock: *Example:* No one to watch the kids so I can go for a walk.

How to Get Past it: Pop the kids into a stroller and we can all walk together. Put on some music and dance in the family room. Put on an aerobics video and let the kids follow along with me.

Roadblock: _____
How to Get Past it: _____

_____

Roadblock: _____
How to Get Past it: _____

_____

Roadblock: _____
How to Get Past it: _____

_____

Roadblock: _____
How to Get Past it: _____

_____

exercises in the sidebar on page 104 to begin your fitness routine and expand your flexibility. In the upcoming sections of this chapter, we will help you use your time study to help you find ways to fit some physical activity into your day, such as climbing the stairs at work or taking 2- or 5-minute walks—perhaps instead of having that cigarette at your coffee break. Think about what would happen if for every cigarette you would have had in the course of a day, you decided to take a walk instead. You'd be much more active. Remember, you don't have to find a single 30- or 45-minute block of time to exercise—those smaller bouts add up.

- *"I'm just too tired to exercise right now."*

Being active can actually give you more energy. Physical activity increases your blood flow and can make you feel upbeat and alert. The more active you are, the more you will increase your stamina. This is especially important for you at this stage because you might feel some fatigue in the first few weeks after you've quit smoking. When you feel tired, try to push yourself a little—you won't regret it.

- *"I don't have exercise equipment and can't afford a gym membership."*

Physical activity does not require gym memberships or expensive classes. It can be done in the settings of your daily life—at home, in the office, or just about anywhere. Some people like to do their physical activity in front of the TV or while listening to music. A great thing about working physical activity into your routines is that you will be setting a wonderful example for the rest of your family. Once they see how great you're doing, they may even want to join you.

- *"I don't know how to exercise."*

You don't need to be an expert to work more activity into your life. You just need to be willing to try. In the next sections, we will help you find ways to transform moments of inactivity—in which you are sitting or not moving around—into more active ones. These might also be moments when you tended to smoke, so you will actually be doing two things at once. Read on for some simple tips on becoming more active that don't require any special skills.

- *"The weather is bad (too hot or too cold)."*
Don't let bad weather stand in your way. If it's too hot or too cold to walk outside, you can always do some heavy housework or take a few trips up and down the stairs. Many towns have shopping malls with special hours for walkers. Mall walking can be a safe and climate-controlled place to walk year-round. Swimming is great for those really hot days, but if you think that is too vigorous an activity for you right now, just walking a couple of laps around the pool can get the blood pumping. On cold winter days, take the kids sledding—walking in the snow is an excellent workout and a couple of trips up the slope can really get your heart rate going.

Setting Goals and Getting Started

Now that you have a better idea of your daily routine and what might stand in the way of becoming more active, try to set some simple goals for yourself. Different methods work for different people, and at this stage you may just want to focus on adding some physical activity at those times when you feel a strong craving to smoke. Be sure to start out safely and gradually and set goals that are realistic—ones that you can really do.

In chapter two (page 46), we asked you some questions

about your health and suggested that you talk to your doctor about becoming more active. Be sure to go back to that section if needed before you start to increase your level of activity.

If you determined that you are ready to get going, set a couple of realistic goals for yourself. The important thing is that you don't rush in too quickly and set yourself up for failure. Staying off cigarettes is a tough thing to do, and for starters, we want you to use physical activity to help you accomplish this goal.

QUICK ACTIVITIES TO GET YOU STARTED

- When going shopping, park farther away from the store than you usually do.
- When watching TV, walk or march in place, or do jumping jacks during commercial breaks.
- Walk around the mall one or more extra times.
- Stretch at various points throughout the day.
- Take the stairs instead of escalators or elevators.
- Do the chair exercises listed below, while at home or at work.

Chair Stretches and Exercises

1. Strengthen your leg muscles by extending your leg out in front of you and hold for 30 seconds. As your leg gets stronger, add 1 pound ankle weights. Do one leg at a time or hold both up together.
2. While seated, slowly point your toes away from your body until you feel some tension and hold the stretch 30 seconds.
3. Slowly rotate your feet clockwise 15 times and then counterclockwise. Rotate your shoulders forward and backward 15 times.
4. If possible, take off your shoes and while sitting try writing the alphabet and numbers with your feet. It's a fun way to get those muscles working.

Look at your time study. For some of those moments of inactivity, try to fill in ways to be more active. For example, if you find yourself sitting at your desk during the day, make a point of getting up once in a while and taking a walk across the office. If you find yourself sitting in front of the TV, try to get up during each commercial break and walk around the house. Or you can try some of the quick activities we suggest on page 104. If you feel that you can do more, try using some of the suggestions in the moderate or vigorous list.

Moderate-Intensity Activities

Regular, vigorous physical activity for at least 30 minutes per day can positively affect your health, especially your weight. Our research has shown, however, that doing moderate-intensity physical activity in bouts of at least 10 minutes and totaling at least 30 minutes a day for 5 days a week or more can help with weight management and physical fitness. If you don't have a 30-minute block of time to be physically active, you can enjoy some of the same benefits by breaking up your physical activity and doing some at different times during the day. If you are struggling to find the time, try fitting in three or four 10- or 15-minute brisk walks throughout the day. Below is a list of moderate-intensity activities for you to try.

- Check your local community center and see what kind of classes they offer. Salsa classes, belly dancing, or self-defense can be fun and are a great way to meet people while being active.

- Garden or do yard work, such as raking the leaves, mowing the lawn, or weeding the garden, or wash your car. These are all physical activities because they involve bending and stretching.

- Get some housework done. Vacuum the carpet, clean windows, scrub the floor.

- Get involved in sports such as volleyball, Frisbee™, or golfing without a cart.

- Walk some laps at your local community pool or sign up for a low-impact water-aerobics class.

- Go dancing.

- Participate in the American Lung Association Asthma Walk in your area. Visit http://www.lungusa.org/asthmawalk/ for details on how to sign up.

- Walk around a museum or take a city walking tour.

- Take a yoga class.

- Take a brisk walk around the neighborhood to see the sun rise or after work to enjoy the sunset.

- Go to the park and fly a kite.

A WORD ABOUT YOGA

Yoga was developed in India about 5,000 years ago to promote unity of the mind, body, and spirit. It is a system of physical activity and fitness that includes a series of poses, postures, and positions. The typical yoga workout is a blend of strength, flexibility, and body awareness exercises. There are many forms of yoga, but the most common is called hatha yoga. Hatha yoga includes all of the basic yoga moves and breathing exercises but doesn't include the religious or spiritual aspects of some the other forms. The general goal of all yoga forms is to increase physical fitness and the ability to maintain positive thoughts and feelings. Classes range from moderately intense to extremely challenging, so make sure to pick one that suits your abilities and fitness level.

Vigorous-Intensity Activities

If you feel up to it, try some of the vigorous physical activities listed below. Be sure to use caution if you are stepping up your routine. Remember, the more active you are, the easier it will be for you to manage your weight.

- Jumping rope can get your blood pumping, increase body awareness, and develop your hand and foot coordination.

- Get a step bench at your local sports store. Most step platforms come with suggested exercises from beginner to more advanced workouts.

- Do some lap swimming at your local community pool.

- Go for a challenging 20-minute bike ride.

- Take an aerobics or dance class, or try karate or kickboxing.

- Give rollerskating a try. In the winter months, ice skating is a great alternative.

- Play tennis or racquetball.

- Go to the YMCA or a gym with a friend and jog next to each other on treadmills.

- Take a bike ride in your neighborhood. Get a group together for a weekly "bike trek" to a nearby park.

- Take a day trip to the beach or a lake and go for a swim.

- Join a sports team at work, or do a 5K run/walk for charity.

ACTION ITEM

Use your time study on page 99 to fill in the worksheet below. If you found that you were inactive for most of your day, use some of the examples on page 104 and try to fit them into your week. If you found that you were already somewhat active, you might want to use more of the tips in the list of moderate-intensity activities on pages 105–106 and try to fit them in on a daily basis. If you feel you can do more, choose from the list of vigorous-intensity activities on page 107. You can pick and choose from all three lists if you like.

Example:

RESULTS OF TIME STUDY

Time Slot	Tasks/Activities/ Smoking?	Physically Active?
7:00 – 9:00 am	Having morning coffee (usually have a cigarette with the coffee)	No
1:00 – 3:00 pm	Sitting at my desk at work (usually take a smoke break at this time)	Yes, took a 10-minute walk.

Time of Day, Activity	How I Am Going To Incorporate Physical Activity
Example: Thursday 7:00 – 9:00 am having morning coffee and cigarette	(for a quick activity) Instead of the cigarette, I'll leave early for work and park further away so I can do a 2-minute walk to the office. Or I'll get off the bus one stop early and walk the rest of the way.

Time of Day, Activity	How I Am Going To Incorporate Physical Activity
Example: Thursday 7:00 – 9:00 am having morning coffee and cigarette	*(for a moderate-intensity activity):* Instead of the cigarette, I'll take a 15-minute brisk walk around the neighborhood before my morning shower.
Example: Monday 1:00 – 3:00 pm, sitting at my desk at work (usually when I take my smoke break)	*(for a quick activity):* Do some stretching exercises. Take a 10-minute walk when I would have had a cigarette break.
	(for a moderate-intensity activity): During my 3:00 pm break I'll try walking up and down the stairs a couple of times.

Now that you have some goals in mind, you can begin. Making small changes in your daily routines can be fun, and you'll see that adding some physical activity to your day can help you get past the urge to smoke. In the next chapter, we'll help you to start thinking about how you can make similar changes in your eating habits.

Above all, remember that you don't need cigarettes! You have already begun to be a nonsmoker. It may not have been easy, but you've taken some great strides toward a much healthier life.

Staying Smoke-free: Making Healthy Eating Choices

6

"*Every time I got a craving for a cigarette, I started to snack on sweets and salty foods such as chips and french fries. I felt like I was addicted to them! But then, I decided to save the chips for after I made it through a week without cigarettes. When the cravings came, I ate fruit, yogurt, or graham crackers. That really helped me get through the cravings.*" (Kathy, age 46)

In the last five chapters, you've been focusing on how to stay off cigarettes in some healthy and creative ways. Maybe you've started to get more physically active or have begun to think about eating better. In any case, you should be proud of yourself for having made it this far. Staying smoke-free is a really tough thing to do, and you have made a lot of progress. Congratulations!

As we've discussed, balancing quitting smoking with getting more physically active and making healthier eating choices can be a challenge. Remember the merry-go-round we discussed earlier—quitting smoking, gaining weight, going back to smoking to lose weight, then quitting again? The best way to get off this merry-go-round is to make quitting smoking your number one priority and to work on managing your weight only to the extent that it does not jeopardize your quitting smoking. So cut yourself some slack, give yourself a pat on the back, and don't get down on yourself if you gain some weight. See if you can use some ideas in this chapter to help you eat healthier while you get used to life without cigarettes.

FOODS THAT BOOST YOUR IMMUNE SYSTEM

Maintaining a healthy, well-functioning immune system is essential to all of us. This is especially important for smokers and ex-smokers for several reasons. First, research shows that prolonged smoking or exposure to tobacco smoke can weaken the body's immune system. Second, research also shows that many smokers' diets don't include enough of the fruits and vegetables that help the immune system. Also, eating right can stave off infection, prevent disease—even reduce the risk of cancer—and help keep you in optimum health.

Like quitting smoking and becoming more physically active, your eating choices are an important part of your health. Healthy eating can reduce your risk for heart disease by helping you control your blood pressure, cholesterol levels, and your weight. The vitamins and minerals in many foods, especially fruits and vegetables, can help improve your health, and studies show that most smokers don't get enough of these nutrients. Healthy eating can also reduce your chances of getting other illnesses such as type 2 diabetes, cancer, gallbladder disease, sleep apnea (when breathing is interrupted during sleep), and osteoarthritis (wearing away of the joints). By eating healthy foods each time you would usually smoke a cigarette, you'll be able to get the nutrients you need and keep away from smoking.

Scientific research shows that you can stimulate your immune system with diet. White blood cells are the front line warriors against infections. Scientific studies have shown that certain foods and nutrients can help increase concentrations of these white blood cells and their potency. Following are some foods that have this beneficial effect on the immune system:

Foods & Nutrients That Stimulate the Immune System

- Yogurt

- Mushrooms

- Citrus fruits

- Onions

- Tomatoes and tomato products (like tomato sauce and tomato paste)

- Garlic

- Beta-carotene: spinach, carrots, sweet potatoes, kale, and pumpkin

- Vitamin C: citrus fruits and their juices, strawberries, kiwi fruit, potatoes, tomatoes

- Vitamin E: plant oils (canola and olive oil, for example)

- Zinc: oysters, crab, turkey, pumpkin, and squash seeds

Remember, the best way to get the nutrients you need is from foods. Daily multi-vitamins are also fine to take. However, high doses of some nutrients (zinc, for example) can actually suppress your own immune system. Before taking individual supplements of vitamins, minerals, or herbs, talk to your doctor or to a registered dietitian for some more personal advice.

At this point, you still may be feeling some of the more negative sensations associated with quitting, such as cravings for sweet, crunchy, or salty foods, stress, lack of energy, boredom, and frustration. Some of these negative feelings can lead you to eat poorly. In fact, after quitting smoking, many people gain weight because of poor eating choices, because extra snacking can become a way of coping with cravings or stress. Plus, without the bad taste of cigarettes in your mouth, food may taste and smell better, which could lead to extra helpings. In this chapter, we'll give you tips for combating these cravings and coping with boredom, stress, and frustration by learning how to snack well and eat in moderation.

Remember, making small habit changes can yield big rewards later. The healthy eating choices you make right now, even the smallest ones, can really add up. Plus, you'll probably find that within a couple of weeks, the cravings will fade away and you will have already started to develop eating habits that can keep you healthy for the rest of your life. If you reach for healthy foods during a craving, before long, you'll crave healthy foods rather than cigarettes.

Getting Encouragement and Cooperation from Family and Friends

As with all regular habits, the people in your life—your friends, family, co-workers—can influence what you do. Eating is a common way of socializing, and many people enjoy spending time together over lunch or dinner, which can make it difficult to maintain a healthy eating style. While some people in your life may have a good influence on your eating habits, others might actually make it harder. They may not mean any harm, but the way in which they approach their eating can have an effect on you.

In chapter eight, we'll help you think more closely about

Things I Can Ask of My Friends and Family to Help Me Make Healthy Eating Choices

- Keep a positive attitude and try to be encouraging, even when I am in a bad mood or struggling.
- Keep the household as stress-free as possible, at least within the first couple of weeks of when I get started.
- Do some physical activity with me, such as walking, so that I'm not tempted to snack as much.
- Listen and talk with me about my progress or my doubts.
- Don't be critical of me when I slip up.
- Be there for me when I am feeling tempted.
- Cook healthy meals with me and help make healthy eating fun.

how social situations affect your eating decisions. For now, start thinking about how your friends and family can support you in trying to make some basic changes to your eating habits. These may be the same people you asked to help you quit smoking or to help with your physical activity goals. Think about what you can ask your family and friends to do to help—from cooking healthy meals with you, to helping you say no to high-calorie foods, to listening when you are feeling sad or frustrated. You might find that your friends and family are watching what they eat and would be happy to have an enthusiastic partner.

Food Diary: Looking at When, Where, and How You Eat

Often people eat without really thinking about what they are putting into their bodies. And usually, what we eat is tied to why we eat—the time of day, how we are feeling, whom we are with, and various other factors. Because our eating habits are part of our everyday life, it can be difficult to identify habits that may not be good for us. For example, now that you have quit smoking, you may tend to eat more often, but don't even realize you are doing it.

In this section, we will ask you to track your eating habits for three or four days so that you can get a better idea of when, where, and how you might make more healthy eating choices. At this stage, you are just starting to gather information about yourself so that you can use it later to set goals for making better eating choices in the future.

Do you notice any patterns in your eating habits? Do you tend to eat more at certain times of the day? Did you notice a relationship between when you eat and your feelings or the urge to smoke? Do you eat more when consuming alcoholic beverages? Are you drinking enough water? We'll return to these questions later when we ask you to use your food diary to set some basic goals for yourself. But first, once you have a better idea of your eating patterns, let's look at what might stand in your way of changing them for the better. In the next section, we'll help you to identify roadblocks to making healthy eating choices and supply you with many tips for how to get past them. This information will also help you when you are ready to set those goals.

ACTION ITEM

Make three or four photocopies of the following worksheet to keep a diary of your eating habits. Try to pick three or four days that include weekdays and those on the weekend. Try to be as accurate as possible, and make sure to keep the worksheets because we will use them later in this chapter.

WORKSHEET: TRACKING YOUR EATING HABITS

- Under the column titled "What and How Much I Ate and Drank," write down what you ate and drank and approximately how much. Don't worry about being too exact; the idea is to get a rough estimate of your food and beverage intake.
- Under the column titled "Other," write down whether you were in a good, normal, or bad mood and whether you felt a craving to smoke. Also indicate if you were with other people or by yourself, and where you were.

Example

Date: January 3		Day of Week: Thursday	
When	**What and How Much I Ate and Drank**	**Feelings**	**Where and With Whom**
7 – 11 am	Coffee with whole milk (usually have a cigarette with the coffee) and two breakfast doughnuts.	Craving a cigarette; had the doughnut instead. Felt anxious.	With my family at home.
3 – 7 pm	Soft drink and bag of potato chips.	Craving a cigarette. Felt normal.	At work, sitting at my desk.

Continued on next page

Adapted from B.H. Marcus & L.H. Forsyth, 2003, *Motivating people to be physically active* (Champaign, IL: Human Kinetics), 103.

Continued from previous page

Worksheet: Tracking Your Eating Habits

Date:		Day of Week:	
When	**What and How Much I Ate and Drank**	**Feelings**	**Where and With Whom**
7 – 11 am			
11 – 3 pm			
3 – 7 pm			
7 – 11 pm			
11 – 3 am			
3 – 7 am			

Overcoming Roadblocks to Healthy Eating

Now that you have quit smoking, you are probably experiencing some roadblocks to staying off cigarettes. Perhaps you are using food as a way to cope with the temptation to go back to smoking. Many ex-smokers have strong urges to eat more or to snack on high-fat and high-calorie foods, especially within the first few weeks after quitting. Perhaps you got used to having something in your mouth and in your hands at certain times of the day and in certain situations. Now that you've quit, you may feel that something's missing, and this feeling may be linked to the times and situations in which you used to smoke. Some of the extra snacking you may be doing might also be linked to feeling sad, frustrated, or stressed. Many people—whether they have ever smoked or not—tend to eat more when they feel low, jittery, or nervous.

As tough as some of these roadblocks are, there are ways to get past them. How? By planning ahead! In this section, we will ask you to identify your roadblocks to healthy eating that are specifically related to having recently quit smoking. Later on, we'll deal with some more general roadblocks to healthy eating. For now, let's focus on keeping you off cigarettes and making sure you are keeping your eating in check.

Key to Overcoming Roadblocks— Anticipation and Cleverness

Earlier, we talked about the importance of anticipating roadblocks and temptations as the key to managing or avoiding them. From your experience over the last few days tracking your eating habits, try to think about what challenges

ACTION ITEM

Make a list of your roadblocks to healthy eating. On the "Roadblock" line, write down something that gets in your way of making more healthy eating choices and choosing healthier alternatives. On the "Anticipate" line, make a note of when and where it tends to happen. On the "How to Get Past it" line, write down a creative solution you can use. Do this for each roadblock you identify.

HEALTHY EATING CHOICES: OVERCOMING ROADBLOCKS

Examples:

Roadblock: Craving for a cigarette and for something sweet.
Anticipate: When or where does it occur?
How to Get Past it: Eat some low-fat frozen yogurt with strawberries on top. Make sure to have fruits on hand or chopped veggies for when I am in a rush.

Roadblock: Now that I am not smoking, I get bored and feel like I want something to do, so I eat.
Anticipate: When or where does it occur?
How to Get Past it: Drink a glass of water every couple of hours. Take a walk, stretch, or do some relaxation exercises when I get the urge to smoke.

Roadblock: _____

Anticipate: _____

How to Get Past it: _____

_____

Roadblock: _____

Anticipate: _____

How to Get Past it: _____

_____

Roadblock: _____

Anticipate: _____

How to Get Past it: _____
_____

Roadblock: _____

Anticipate: _____

How to Get Past it: _____
_____

may lie ahead for you. If you can anticipate and think cleverly about ways you can cope with your challenges, you should be able to get past them. Below are some of the most common roadblocks for ex-smokers trying to make healthy eating choices. Tips follow for how to get past each one. Even if some of these don't apply to you, you can still use the tips as starting points for your own strategies.

- **Roadblock:** Increased feelings of hunger and overeating.

  "After quitting, I started feeling hungry more often and tended to eat more, especially at those times when I used to smoke."

  How to Get Past It: Know if you are really hungry. Slow down. Eat balanced meals.

  Knowing If You are Really Hungry. A point to ponder as you work on making healthy eating choices is the difference between hunger and appetite. Hunger is based on your body's need for food to give it energy. Appetite, on the other hand, is when you eat based on your emotions or other factors like time of day. Sometimes our body gives us signs of physical hunger, such as a rumbling stomach or fatigue or irritability. But other times, the sights and smells around us trigger us to eat, even though we really aren't hungry. Do you notice any patterns in your food diary? Maybe you tended to eat when you were frustrated or stressed. Maybe you ate more when you were bored and irritable. People commonly lose control over their eating at these times and frequently overeat or eat when they aren't really hungry. Your eating style is part of a system of habits just as your smoking habit was. Sometimes these habits have become so ingrained that we don't even realize what we are doing.

Next time you open the refrigerator, ask yourself the following questions: Am I really hungry? When was the last time I ate? Would a snack do, or do I need a full meal? Make a list of five tasks you'll do before eating anything to see if you are really hungry—you may not want a snack when you are done. For example, try taking a quick (2- or 5-minute) walk (or longer), wash your face, stretch for a couple of minutes, file or paint your nails, or call a friend.

Slowing Yourself Down. In addition to considering whether you are really hungry before you eat, you may also want to find ways to slow down while in the process of eating. Try to chew your food more slowly. Rest your fork and knife between bites. Give your body 20 minutes to digest the meal before you decide to go for a second helping. Try drinking water throughout each meal. It will slow you down and fill you up. After dinner, don't linger at the table; get up and clean the kitchen or do some physical activity.

Eating a Balanced Meal. You can also satisfy increased feelings of hunger by eating more balanced meals. Having a balanced eating style may take a little more planning than having some healthy snacks on hand. But you can work up to it. Start by trying to eat more of the kinds of foods that are good for your health—the Food Guide Pyramid on page 48 can help.

As we saw in chapter two, nutritionists recommend eating

at least 5 servings a day of vegetables and fruits. If you have a hard time managing two or three, don't panic. Instead, pat yourself on the back every time you choose to eat a piece of fruit. Keep building on your successes and keep in mind your first priority is not smoking. If having a little candy every day is what you need to get through your smoking urges, then go ahead and have

> ### CALORIES DO COUNT
>
> Eating foods like whole grains, fruits, vegetables and moderate amounts of lean meats and fish are great, but overeating applies to healthy food, too. It's simple —eating too much of any food will make you gain weight. Chances are you won't consume enough fruits and vegetables for this to be a problem, but watch your serving sizes when you're eating carbohydrates, even if they are made from whole grains since they can add inches to your waistline.

it. As the nicotine cravings start to go away, then you can focus on ridding yourself of your candy habit.

- **Roadblock:** Eating because of boredom, stress, or depression.

"I eat when I am feeling down or bored or craving a cigarette because eating comforts me."

How to Get Past It: Use physical activity and healthy snacking.

Many people use food as a kind of pick-me-up or eat when there isn't anything else to do. Maybe you noticed from your food diary that you tend to eat more when you are feeling depressed or when you're in a bad mood. Part of overcoming this kind of roadblock is identify your eating style. Once you know why you eat, you can figure out ways to substitute unnecessary snacking with more healthy choices. For women, menstruation can be a particularly difficult time. Many women say that they feel sad, anxious, or tired, and usually have more cravings for salts or sweets at certain times during their menstrual cycle. Try to fill your refrigerator with fruit and your cabinet with low-fat popcorn or pretzels and other snacks that can satisfy your taste for something sweet and salty.

◆ **Roadblock:** The time bind

"I don't have the time to count calories or worry about what I eat. Smoking was just an easier way to keep the weight off."

How to Get Past it: Make alternative food choices and plan ahead.

We all say we don't have enough time. But what we really mean is that we've got so much to do already that we don't have enough energy to give attention to another task. Making healthy eating choices does involve some effort and planning, but there are ways to eat well that don't require too much preparation . When you do have some extra time, cut up some vegetables or make a fruit salad for when you need a snack. Having healthier foods in front of you will help you make healthier choices. When you go grocery shopping, go to the produce section first. Keep a bowl of fruit in an obvious place in your kitchen so that you can grab a piece when you are really busy. When you are going to work, pack some healthy snacks so you don't run out and buy a candy bar. And again, if the candy bar is what you really want, try to be strategic about when you eat one. Turn it into a special occasion rather than a habit.

Reach for healthier alternatives for a quick and easy way to eat better instead of trying to cook elaborate meals or counting calories. Below are several suggestions for doing this. Keep in mind, though, that fat-free and sugar-free foods still have calories—and more of any food equals weight gain.

What are your roadblocks to healthy eating? The Action Item on page 122 will help you devise a strategy for your healthy new lifestyle.

Setting Goals for Healthy Eating

Now that you have an idea of your eating patterns and the roadblocks that might get in the way, you can use some of that information to set some simple goals. When setting them, remember that changing your eating habits takes some patience and planning. Usually, we want to change everything at once, especially when it comes to weight management and improving our appearance. But if you start out slowly and work on two or three of the habits that you want to change, success will come more quickly and last longer. You might choose to set a goal to give up the bag of chips you crave from time to time and instead have a healthier alternative. You could try to eat more fruits and vegetables in general. Whatever it may be, make your goals doable, simple, and easy to achieve.

Try to set goals that are clear. Instead of saying, "I'll cut down on the sweets" make your goal more defined, like, "The next time I crave something sweet, I'll have some strawberries with low-fat yogurt instead." Or, rather than say "I am going to eat less cheese," try to locate specific times when you can cut back on cheese, such as not adding it to your hamburger, baked potato, or broccoli.

You've made a great start toward a healthier lifestyle. In the next couple of chapters, we'll show you how to create a more balanced eating plan and help you use healthy eating to keep up your good work and get through your first couple of months of being a nonsmoker. Get started on your goals and enjoy the changes you are making. The smallest changes can really change your life, and reaching your goals will surely build your confidence. You are staying smoke-free and managing your weight—a job well done!

Healthier Alternatives to Sweets and Desserts

USE LOWER-FAT DAIRY FOODS
- Try using sherbet, sorbet, or fruit ices instead of ice cream.
- Try low-fat frozen yogurt; low-calorie Fudgsicles™, Popsicles™, or frozen juice bars.
- Make puddings or custards with fat-free milk.

USE LOWER-FAT BAKED GOODS
- Angel food cake, gingersnaps, fig bars, animal crackers, graham crackers, apple and strawberry bars.
- Non-fat cakes and cookies.
- Try to doctor up your high-fat desserts by removing something from them. Try cutting the crust off the pie, get ice cream without toppings, order desserts without whipped cream.

CHOOSE FRUIT FOR DESSERT
- Top your frozen yogurt with berries or other kind of fruits to sweeten it up.
- Eat fruit with gelatin.
- Blend fruits into a fruit drink.

SOME OTHER SWEETS
- hard candy, licorice, jelly beans, and gum drops.

Healthier Alternatives for Other Foods

High-Fat Food Choices	Lower-Fat Alternatives
BEEF rib roasts, hamburger, brisket, short ribs, rib eye, sirloin, T-bone steaks	**BEEF** extra lean ground beef, flank steak, sirloin tip, round steak
CHEESE cheddar, American, bleu, Swiss	**CHEESE** part skim mozzarella, parmesan, low-calorie Swiss
CEREAL Granola	**CEREAL** oatmeal, Cornflakes™, Cheerios™, Shredded Wheat™, Puffed Rice™
PORK bacon, spareribs, shoulder cuts, sausages, lunch meats	**PORK** loin chops, fresh/smoked ham, pork tenderloin
SEAFOOD breaded or fried	**SEAFOOD** grilled, broiled, or baked
CHICKEN with skin, grilled	**CHICKEN** without skin, broiled
POTATOES french fried, au gratin	**POTATOES** oven-fried, baked
SNACK FOODS potato chips, cheese curls, tortilla chips	**SNACK FOODS** unbuttered popcorn, pretzels, rice cakes

ACTION ITEM

SETTING SOME SIMPLE GOALS

Write down your goals on the blanks below. When setting goals, use the Food Guide Pyramid and your food diary. Ask yourself which food categories you are already doing well with and where there's room for improvement. For example, you might be eating too many foods from the tip of the Pyramid but not eating enough vegetables. If eating vegetables or fruits is a challenge for you, brainstorm about how you can fit them into your day (for example, add raisins to your cereal or some spinach to your sandwich). Look at your food diary to better understand your feelings when you eat. Remember to anticipate the times when you want to make the changes. Make plans for how you will make healthy eating choices at those times. Remember to use physical activity as a way to get past cravings when you aren't really hungry and want to delay a snack.

Example:

WHAT I WANT TO CHANGE

1. I don't eat enough fruits or vegetables.
2. I eat too many sweets.
3. I feel like when I get a craving to smoke I lose control of my eating and binge on fattening foods.

HOW I AM GOING TO CHANGE IT

Time and Place	New Behavior
Lunch at work	Eat fruit instead of cookies and cake
Dinner at home	Eat at least one vegetable
Cravings for snacks or cigarettes during the day	Go for a 5-minute walk

WHAT I WANT TO CHANGE

1. _____

2. _____

3. _____

HOW I AM GOING TO CHANGE IT

Time and Place	New Behavior

Three Weeks to Six Months after Quitting

7

Congratulations on making it through the first three weeks of being a nonsmoker. You should feel really good about yourself right now. You have made tremendous strides toward achieving a difficult and important goal. You should feel confident that, having come this far, you can make it all the way to a long life without cigarettes. But don't let your guard down —you will still experience strong urges to smoke over the next couple of weeks. Keep anticipating those tough spots and managing them. Be confident, stay smart, and keep up the good work.

Have you been working on the goals you set for healthy eating and physical activity in chapters five and six? Have you made it through some roadblocks? Let's start building on your successes and going to the next level. In this chapter, we'll help you set new goals for becoming more active and developing a healthy eating style. If you haven't started to work on these areas yet, try reading through chapters five and six to get started. Physical activity and healthy eating can help you stay smoke-free and manage your weight—indeed, they are key ingredients for your health and overall well-being.

We'll also provide you with some additional coping strategies for staying off cigarettes, this time focusing more on the emotional challenges of staying smoke-free and keeping a positive outlook. These strategies are particularly important for overcoming frustration, stress, or low mood and can also help you cope with social situations that might challenge your resolve.

CONTINUED USE OF NICOTINE REPLACEMENT PRODUCT

By about 2 to 3 months after you quit, you may begin to cut down on your nicotine replacement. You may want to do this slowly. The amount of nicotine in patches, inhalers, gum, and other nicotine replacement products is low enough that you don't have to worry about using them a little longer than you may have originally planned. It's more important, however, that you not stop using nicotine replacement too soon. Sometimes users begin to feel confident, quit the product, and then relapse. Make sure you use the nicotine replacement until you are certain you can go without. Most people use nicotine replacement at least 4 to 6 weeks, many up to six months. There's no magic number. The critical thing is to use it long enough so that when you cut back, you don't find yourself with increased urges. Also, keep some of the nicotine replacement with you after you stop using it. This may help you deal with unanticipated urges.

Stepping It Up: Setting New Goals for Physical Activity and Healthy Eating

Focus on: Physical Activity

Now that you've started to do some 2- or 5-minute walks throughout your day, or started a yoga or low-impact aerobics class, let's try to make your physical activity regimen more interesting. If you feel you aren't ready for any changes right now, just review this section and come back to it when you feel as if you might be ready for something new. If you haven't been working on physical activity at all, why not go back to chapter five and give it a try? You might find it can really help you stay smoke-free and minimize any weight you may gain. But if you feel that you are ready to test out some new activities or increase the ones you are doing now, let's get you started.

A WORD ABOUT SAFETY: PREVENTING INJURY

With any sort of physical activity, it's important that you build up to it and not do too much too soon. With a gradual approach, you'll be strengthening your muscles and stretching your tendons slowly, which can help you to avoid injury. You can avoid injury by stretching before any physical activity. Knee injuries are common injuries for people getting active, so you may especially want to focus on stretching the muscles above your knees and those on the back of your legs. You can find more information on exercising properly in *Active Living Every Day* by S.N. Blair, A.L. Dunn, B.H. Marcus, R.A. Carpenter, and P. Jaret. Champaign, IL: Human Kinetics, 2001.

- *Try doing your physical activity at different times of the day.*
  If you find yourself getting bored by walking up and down the stairs, try a different time of day. Maybe you walk in the mornings, and could try walking in the afternoon instead, or doing both. If you are taking a 10- or 15-minute walk in the morning, try switching to the evening to enjoy the sunset. Shuffle your schedule to spice up your routine.

- *Try doing all of your exercise at once.*
  Maybe you can do a 20-minute walk instead of two 10-minute ones, or even better, walk for a full half hour. This

ACTION ITEM

MY PHYSICAL ACTIVITY SCHEDULE

Now that you may have started to add 2-, 5-, and 10-minute walks to your day, make yourself a physical activity schedule. You can use it to figure out where you can fit in some more activity and make it a regular part of your day. Start by filling out the first two columns, indicating the amount of time you spend on each physical activity you are currently doing.

Example:

Day of the Week	Time Slot	My Current Physical Activity	What I Am Going To Add
Monday	7 – 9 am	walk for 10 minutes	
	4 – 5 pm	walk for 15 minutes	
Saturday	7 – 9 am	not active at this time	

Day of the Week	Time Slot	My Current Physical Activity	What I Am Going To Add
Monday			
Tuesday			
Wednesday			
Thursday			
Friday			
Saturday			
Sunday			

might enable you to walk somewhere that you haven't been before or have only driven to. Over a 30-minute span of time, your heart rate will have a chance to increase more steadily, and you may start to build up a sweat. This means that you will be doing moderate-intensity physical activity and that is the kind of activity that can help you burn calories, which in turn can help you manage your weight.

- *Finding something you like to do.*

Take a week and try different types of physical activities. Maybe you've always been curious about yoga, karate, or jazz dancing, but had trouble getting started. Now that you've been walking a couple of days a week, maybe you're ready for a low-impact aerobics class. Classes are great

ACTION ITEM

Now that you have some ideas for how to intensify your physical activity routine, go back to the chart on page 139 and fill in the last column. Here is an example of what it might look like:

Example:

Day of the Week	Time Slot	My Current Physical Activity	What I Am Going To Add
Monday	7 – 9 am	walk for 10 minutes	increase to 15 minutes
	4 – 5 pm	walk for 15 minutes	increase to 20 minutes
Saturday	7 – 9 am	not active at this time	take a low-impact aerobics class at the YMCA

because usually they don't cost too much and can be a wonderful way to meet new people who share the same interests. If attending a class is too much of a burden on your time, try a videotape from your local library, bookstore, or grocery store.

You might try starting a new hobby that involves physical activity. Gardening can be fun and relaxing and you can grow your own fresh vegetables to eat. If you live in the city, you could join a community garden, which will help you be more active and make your city more beautiful. There may be some sports teams in your area for people in your age group. Joining a local softball, soccer, or basketball team is another great way to meet new people or spend time with friends who also want to be active.

Focus on: Healthy Eating

Now that you've set some new goals for physical activity, let's do the same for healthy eating. We'll start by looking at your progress in achieving the goals you set in chapter six, and then we'll add to them. If you find that you aren't ready for any changes right now, just review this section and you can come back to it when you are ready.

Before you get started on setting goals, review the information on pages 128–129. It will give you some new ideas for how to eat healthier when you are eating out. Maintaining a healthy eating style can be difficult if you eat out often, but it's not impossible. Try using some of the tips on eating out when setting new goals for yourself.

Eating Out and Making Healthy Eating Choices

Eating out is a common event for most people. In fact, did you know that more than 50 percent of American meals are now eaten outside the home? When eating out, it is sometimes difficult to identify exactly what you are eating. You may know the basic food item, but there may be a host of other ingredients you are not aware of. Sometimes foods that sound healthy, such as soups or salads, are prepared in ways that make them high in fat and calories. Most restaurants do have low-fat menu choices, but you will need to know how to identify them and to ask for more information. You may also want to try eating out less. Preparing your own food can be a lot of fun. Sometimes it's just the right therapy for when you are bored or feeling low—and it can be a great new project as you look for things to fill the time once taken up by smoking. Below are some tips on how to watch what you are eating when you dine out.

- **Make a List.** Make a list of restaurants that have lower-calorie options. This may mean choosing places that grill or poach their seafood and chicken dishes as opposed to frying them, or places that have "healthy choice" menus. This way, when you are planning a night out, you will already have some good suggestions that can accommodate your goal to eat healthy foods.

- **Be Aware of Portions**. When eating out, be aware of portions. Often, restaurant-size portions are larger than those that you would make at home. Try to get an idea of the portion size before you order. You might consider ordering from the appetizer menu or splitting a main entrée with someone else. In some restaurants, meals are served "family style." In this case, you will need to be careful to take only the portion you need. If it becomes difficult, practice some of those tips in chapter six (page 124) about how to slow yourself down.

• *Make Low-Fat Requests.* In addition to asking about portion size, ask your waitperson to explain how your order is made. Don't be shy about asking. You have a right to know. Here are some examples of low- and high-calorie ways of preparing foods. When looking at the menu, watch out for these terms:

Low-calorie Prep	High-calorie Prep
Steamed	Buttered
Broiled	Pan-fried, fried, or crispy
In its own juice	Escalloped
Poached	Au gratin
Garden fresh	Creamed
Grilled	In its own gravy

• *Make Changes at the Table.*
  – Leave butter or margarine off dinner rolls.
  – Politely move the bread basket away from you.
  – Trim the fat off meat and the skin off chicken.
  – Keep water close by and drink it often.

ACTION ITEM

HEALTHY EATING GOALS

Use the worksheet below to work on your goals. Copy the goals you set and how you planned to work on them from page 131 onto the worksheet below in columns one and two. Indicate your progress for each goal in column three. If you haven't met the goal to your

1 Something I Wanted to Change	**2** How I Worked to Change it
I don't eat enough fruits or vegetables.	I am going to eat one serving of vegetables with dinner at least once a week.
I eat too many sweets.	Each time I feel a craving to smoke or eat sweets, I am going to eat a piece of fruit.
I tend to eat more unhealthy foods when eating out with friends.	I am going to make a list of restaurants with healthy menu options and suggest we go to them.
I feel like when I get a craving I lose control of my eating and binge on high-calorie foods.	I am going to take a walk next time I find myself in the middle of a binge.

satisfaction, list some things that you can do to reach it in column four. If you feel like you've met your goal and made it a part of your eating habits, use column four to list some ways to build on that success. There are some blank spaces at the bottom of the chart to set some new goals for yourself. Please use additional paper if necessary.

3 How I Am Doing	**4** What I Can Do to Reach My Goal
Met this goal. Added string beans, corn, and broccoli to my dinners.	Add another serving of these and other vegetables to my lunches and dinners.
Need to keep working on this.	Make fruit more available. Keep a fruit bowl on the kitchen table.
My friends and I are eating at places on my list, but I need to watch my portions.	I am going to start ordering from the appetizer list and eat a light salad if I am still hungry.
Am taking the walks, but could do more.	Keep doing what I am doing but try a little harder. Chew gum to offset the craving.

More Coping Strategies for Staying Smoke-free

Even though you've made it this far, you should still be on guard because your roadblocks can be persistent. Physical activity and healthy eating can do wonders for your effort to stay off cigarettes, but the cravings may not have gone away completely and maybe you found yourself in some tempting situations that you hadn't anticipated. Maybe you lapsed once or twice and don't feel completely confident yet. The following are some extra strategies to keep you positive as you continue to work on staying smoke-free and managing your weight.

THE "I'M HOME FREE" RELAPSE

Maybe you've done this before, or maybe you know others who have. It's been about three weeks since your last cigarette and things have been going well. You are feeling confident. In fact, although it hasn't been easy by any means, it hasn't been as tough as you expected, so you are really feeling in control of your former smoking habit.

You meet some friends for dinner or go to a party where others are smoking. It's after dinner, you're feeling relaxed and think, "A cigarette would really taste good right now. I feel in control, so I'll just make a rule with myself that I only smoke after dinner when I'm out with friends." Two days later you're buying cigarettes by the carton and calling all your friends for dinner dates!

There are two important lessons here. The first is that even though you are feeling confident and in control, you need to keep your guard up and watch for temptations that may sneak up on you. Second, you probably need to recognize that, in the future, it will be easier for you not to smoke at all than to try to manage the occasional cigarette. Why? Because the occasional cigarette forces you to go through much of the whole quitting process again. *Remember, it's easier to have none than one.*

Positive Self-Talk

You already know that quitting smoking requires confidence, creativity, and a "stick with it" attitude. But sometimes life throws curve balls and it's hard to keep a positive attitude when you feel as if you're always striking out. Make sure that you are not expecting too much. Reward yourself from time to time. Treat yourself when you are down or frustrated or you find that you are simply running out of enthusiasm. Your rewards list on pages 72–73 can give you some ideas when you're looking for a little pick-me-up.

When you experience feelings of self-doubt and frustration or are trying to talk yourself out of doing something that is good for you, try what's called "positive self-talk." Positive self-talk is saying positive things to yourself that can help you to think more clearly, stay calm, and focus. It can also help you when you feel depressed or are in a bad mood. Negative self-talk works the opposite way. It can turn a simple challenge into a major event, and weaken your ability to handle tough situations. This is especially true when you are faced with a roadblock or a strong temptation to smoke.

The same goes for physical activity and healthy eating. You can easily talk yourself out of going for your morning walk, citing any number of excuses. It's always okay to take a break now and then, but don't let negative self-talk become a habit that hampers your efforts to get more active. Countering the negative with positive self-talk may be all you need to get out the door, onto the sidewalk, and walking. Positive self-talk can keep you from having an extra helping at the breakfast table, even when you are having a strong craving to smoke.

Below are some examples of both kinds of self-talk. Read these over and add a couple of your own in the extra spaces. If you find yourself slipping into negative self-talk, come back to this page and remind yourself that there is a different way to look at it. You may even want to practice saying some of these statements to yourself or do some role-playing with your quitting coach or partner.

Negative Self-Talk	Positive Self-Talk
"Just one cigarette won't hurt."	*"I am a nonsmoker. I don't need a cigarette."*
"I'm too tired to walk right now."	*"Taking a walk will make me feel energized and ready to start my day."*
"One more doughnut won't hurt."	*"I'm not really hungry and I've been doing so well in watching what I eat."*
"I thought I had it beat, but right now I feel that I want a cigarette so much, it's like I smoked my last one an hour ago."	*"It's not easy yet—that's what I know to expect, but I've made a lot of progress and am getting through most of the time without too much trouble."*

The following are some more general positive statements that can be applied to staying smoke-free and to your efforts to get more active or make healthy eating choices. Add one or more of your own in the empty spaces below:

- *"This is hard, but it only gets easier."*
- *"I have done a lot of difficult things in my life. I can certainly do this."*
- *"This is what I really want."*
- *"My health is really important so getting to the point where I don't miss cigarettes anymore is worth the extra expense. It's worth asking a favor of my friend(s)…it's worth cutting myself some slack at work."*
- _____
- _____

Benefits of Being a Nonsmoker

You already know the many benefits of quitting smoking, but let's go over some of the benefits you have experienced in the last couple of weeks. You may have noticed that your clothes and hair no longer smell of cigarettes, or that the walk up the stairs got a little easier. Reminding yourself of the advantages of being a non-smoker can keep you motivated through times of doubt or frustration. The following is an exercise you might try when you need some positive reinforcement.

These positive experiences might be mixed in with some negative ones. You are likely to still experience cravings and may even feel some nostalgia for the days when you used to have a cigarette with your morning coffee or evening glass of wine. Remind yourself that you are doing the best thing you

---

ACTION ITEM

In the worksheet below, fill in some of the benefits of quitting smoking that you've started to experience now that you have quit.

BENEFITS I HAVE ALREADY NOTICED

1. **Example:** My clothes don't smell like cigarettes anymore.

2. **Example:** I don't breathe heavily when I walk up the stairs.

3. **Example:** I don't have to stand outside in the cold to have a cigarette during my lunch break.

4. _____

5. _____

6. _____

7. _____

can do for your health, and that to live a healthier life is what you really want. In the worksheet below, remind yourself of the many benefits of being a nonsmoker. Go back to pages 27–29 if you need a refresher on the positive effects of quitting to which you can look forward.

STAYING MOTIVATED: YOUR LIFE SAVINGS

By quitting smoking you are literally saving your life. But you are also saving money. The cost of cigarettes has increased dramatically in recent years with many states imposing high taxes on cigarettes and other tobacco products. If you used to smoke a pack a day, you're now saving over $2,000 a year by not smoking. That's enough for a wonderful vacation or can be a great contribution toward your child's college fund. When trying to stay motivated, think of all the money you are saving.

I AM LOOKING FORWARD TO...

1. **Example:** Saving enough money in my cigarette fund to go on a vacation.
2. **Example:** Having more energy and being more physically active.
3. **Example:** Living a longer, healthier life with less risk of heart attack, stroke, cancer, and other serious illnesses.

4._____

5._____

6._____

7._____

Assertive Communication and Saying No

Another important part of keeping a positive attitude is learning how to deal with social situations that can make it difficult for you to not smoke. Remember, quitting smoking is an important step for your well-being. While many people will want to help you, some might make it more difficult, whether they know it or not. This is especially true for people who don't know you and offer you a cigarette, or others who don't know that you quit smoking. You may also find that some smokers just haven't recognized how lethal smoking is and think they're being a good friend by offering you a cigarette. The key to overcoming this roadblock is first knowing how to say no. There are many ways to do this, but the best way is to keep a positive tone and say no with confidence and grace.

This advice applies to situations in which people are not being as sensitive as you'd like them to be. Negative interactions can pull you back into smoking. But you needn't deal with negative interactions in a negative manner. Communication is a two-way street. Try to keep it positive, for both of you. This means learning and practicing effective communication and keeping an upbeat tone.

In this section, we'll give you some tools for building your confidence in dealing with social situations that might tempt you to smoke. Learning how to say no and responding with a positive tone when someone offers you a cigarette can keep you firm in your decision to not smoke and can prevent stressful situations.

Saying No

Saying no to cigarettes is one of the most important ways you can stay smoke-free. There are many ways to say it and the more you say it, the easier it will become. The key is striking a balance between being firm and keeping it light. Different situations will call for different responses. The one constant thing, however, is that you be sure to stay calm. It might be more fun than you think. No is such a simple word, but it can have a considerable effect on your life. Saying no to a cigarette is a way of saying yes to yourself. It is a way to nurture and take care of yourself. Think of all the effort you have put into quitting smoking. A little no can go a long way in keeping it that way.

Below are some examples of different ways you might say no when someone offers you a cigarette:

- Simple and straightforward: *"Thanks, but I would rather not. I quit."*

- Nice, but firm: *"Thanks, but I quit smoking. If you wouldn't mind, please don't offer me a cigarette again."*

- Humorous: *"I'm sorry I can't. I am training for the Olympics and my coach said it wouldn't be good for me."*

Keep in mind that saying no applies to physical activity and healthy eating as well. Sticking to your plan to go for an evening walk can be difficult when your friends want to go for an after-work drink. Sometimes it's a tough call, but learning how to say "no" means protecting the time you set aside to get more active. As for healthy eating, sometimes saying no can be awkward when people offer you something to eat, especially if they are only an acquaintance or you find yourself in a formal situation. But you can still say no politely. Some people, on the other hand, tend to be a bit pushy, and with them, you might need to be a little firmer.

Being Assertive

In trying to keep your communication positive, be sure to maintain a balance and stay upbeat. Generally speaking, there are three ways you can respond in difficult situations with other people. Consider how you might react if a friend or co-worker says something like, "You are so hard to deal with right now, I liked you better when you were smoking."

◆ Aggressive Reaction: *"How dare you try to tempt me. You're not a friend. You don't care about me."*

This kind of reaction can make you feel as if you've lost control over your emotions. This can result in a strong urge to smoke. It also draws attention to you and away from what you really want to emphasize, the fact that you are trying to quit smoking. You want to stay focused on your objective, not get caught in an argument.

◆ Passive Reaction: *You stay silent and become cranky.*

Lack of action can make you feel a loss of self-respect and decrease your confidence. You may think, "Who cares, I might as well have a cigarette."

◆ Assertive Reaction: *"It's hard to quit and maybe I'm making things a bit hard on others as I try to figure out how to live without cigarettes. But it's really important for me and I need to stick with it. Maybe we can discuss ways to work out some compromises."*

In this situation, you took control, explained your position, and directly asked for what you wanted. You also kept the focus on your objectives, by letting go of whether or not you were cranky, so you could stay focused on what's important to you. You respected the other person's feelings, but also respected your own as well. You offered to cooperate with the other person, agreeing to compromise, not giving up your needs in order to please someone else. If you choose to react assertively, you'll feel good about yourself, and will have avoided a potentially dangerous trigger to smoking.

In the following Action Item, practice some of the assertive responses you might use when faced with a negative interaction.

ACTION ITEM

Write down and practice some assertive ways that you can respond when someone challenges you or makes it hard for you to not smoke. Maybe you've already had some of these experiences. Draw from them to plan for the next time.

Example

Situation: *"When I told my friend I was going to stop smoking, she said, "Yeah, you've tried to do that a couple times before…"*

My Response: *"Sure, I went back to smoking before. But this time I learned a lot more about my smoking habit and did some planning. I am really trying to make this time different."*

Situation: _____

My Response: _____

_____

Situation: _____

My Response: _____

_____

Parties and Other Social Occasions

In general, social situations can be a trigger for wanting a cigarette. In chapter four, we suggested you avoid social occasions where you know people will be smoking because they could make it difficult for you to stay smoke-free. Now that you are past the three-week mark, you may want to try a party or social gathering, or at least start to plan what you will do when the opportunity arises. Maybe you already went to one and something triggered you to smoke, even though you were feeling good about having quit. This is perfectly understandable, especially in the first few weeks after quitting when it is so hard to say no. But you want to start thinking seriously about how to get through social situations without having a cigarette.

Before you take the plunge, try to assess if you are really ready to go to that social gathering. If you have been craving a cigarette all day, but have been holding on and not having one, you might think twice about going to a party. Other times, you may be celebrating your nonsmoking status. This might be a good time to try a social gathering and see how you do. (But remember to beware of the "I'm home free" relapse.) The important thing is to be honest with yourself before entering a potentially tough situation. Below is an exercise that you can do to help you decide if you are really ready:

Am I Really Ready?

Put a check in the Yes or No column. When you are finished, add up the number of checks in each column.

Questions	Yes	No
Have I recently had a lapse?		
Am I feeling sad, stressed out, frustrated, or in a bad mood?		
Have I been thinking about smoking all day?		
Do I have trouble saying no?		
Will there be people there who may pressure me to smoke?		
Total:		

If you answered yes to 2 or more questions, you may want to reconsider going to a party with smokers. If you answered no to at least 3 of the questions and think you are ready, you should still plan for the party ahead of time. Try to anticipate what may happen at the party that might put you at risk for a relapse. Think about who will be there. What will happen and when? Will there be dancing that will give you lots of opportunity for having fun and focusing your attention on things other than missing a cigarette? Or, will the party consist of folks standing around, talking, drinking, snacking—would this make it harder for you? Practicing saying no can help, but you also might want to find some other strategies for temptations.

For example, you might want to plan on going with someone who you know is supportive of your efforts. Perhaps you can stay in a room or area where you know smokers will not be congregating. If you think the toughest time will be while people are having drinks before dinner, arrive late. Maybe the toughest time will be after dinner when the party is dragging on, people are getting tired, and you might be feeling bored or vulnerable. Leave early. Anticipate how the party will challenge you and come up with specific plans for coping with those challenges.

Below are some tips for how to make specific plans for social situations that might trigger you to smoke. You may still need to practice some avoidance from time to time, but here you'll develop some great coping strategies for when you decide you are ready.

- *Get Support Ahead of Time.* Make sure that a friend or family member will be available if an emergency situation arises and you need to call someone. Keep his or her phone number with you and call if you need a voice telling you that you don't really need a cigarette. Maybe you can bring your quitting coach for support. You might also tell your friends who will be there that you may need their encouragement during the course of the evening.

- *Try Your New Self On.* If you meet new people at the gathering, try out your new identity by telling them that you are an ex-smoker. It might give you something to talk about if the conversation runs dry and you may make some new friends if they too are trying to quit smoking or have recently become a nonsmoker.

- *Try Not Drinking.* If the social occasion is one where people will be drinking alcohol, consider abstaining for now. You may want to try not drinking for the first couple of parties or gatherings that you attend. Alcohol can significantly increase your desire to smoke and can take away your ability to make sound decisions.

A WORD ABOUT ALCOHOL

Alcohol is an addictive substance and drinking can have negative effects on your health. Studies show that smokers tend to consume greater amounts of alcoholic beverages than do non-smokers. *Alcohol will increase your urge to smoke.* Try the following alternatives: flavored soda water, club soda with lime or lime juice, "virgin" cocktails such as a Bloody Mary or a daiquiri (watch out for the calories on these!), or alcohol-free wine or beer. Think about what alcoholic drinks are associated with smoking in your mind. Maybe there's a type or flavor that, for you, just wouldn't go with smoking. If so, try it, but also remember that if you have too much, you'll lower your guard and put yourself at risk for a smoking relapse.

- *Bring a Survival Pack.* Be smart and prepare for road-blocks ahead of time by bringing hard candy or chewing gum for coping with cravings. Make sure that you have the phone number of your quitting coach and that your reasons for quitting are safely stowed in your purse or wallet. Don't be ashamed to make a phone call or whip out your list to remind yourself why you are quitting and how important it is to you. You can bring other quitting aids as well, such as a rubber band to fidget with and keep your hands busy.

* ***Be Prepared to Take a Walk.*** If the temptation to smoke starts to overwhelm you, be prepared to take a walk or leave the party if you have to. At least you gave it a try, and your friends should understand why you had to leave.

* ***Tell People You've Quit.*** Tell the people you meet at the party that you've quit smoking. If you are feeling a little shaky but really want to get through it without a cigarette, you are likely to get some encouragement.

Now you're just about prepared for any situation that could make you smoke again and you've reinforced all those great lessons you learned in earlier chapters in this book. By gaining the support of your friends and family, planning ahead, and setting goals appropriate to your lifestyle, you set the stage for a sustained program of health that can help you stay smoke-free and manage your weight both in the short and long run. This is the healthy new you we've been talking about!

Six Months and After: The Healthy New You

8

"My Quit Day was the same as my wedding day. It was one of the happiest days of my life. We really want to have kids and now that I am smoke-free and working on my health, I feel much more confident about getting pregnant and starting a family to go along with the healthy new me!" (Anna, age 26)

Now that you've made it past the first six months of quitting smoking, we can finally ask: How does it feel to be a nonsmoker? By now, you're likely to have experienced many of the benefits of quitting smoking and there are still some more to look forward to. If you've been working on getting more physically active, you probably have more energy, and don't have those really strong cravings that at first seemed impossible to satisfy. Plus, you are no longer a slave to your habit. You took control. You really did it.

You've been setting a great example for the people around you. You've shown your friends and family that quitting smoking can be done and that it can really make a difference in your life. By staying smoke-free, you're decreasing your risk of coronary heart disease, stroke, cancer, COPD (Chronic Obstructive Pulmonary Disease), and other serious illnesses, and are lengthening your life. You're helping to create a healthier environment for other people, especially those with whom you live and whose health may have been endangered by secondhand smoke. In short, you've shown yourself and the people in your life the value of a healthy lifestyle and how it can enrich your life.

In this chapter, we'll review some of the lessons and strategies you've learned to stay smoke-free for good and manage your weight. As we said in chapter one, these are lifelong lessons that are part of the overall picture of your health. So keep them in mind as you keep up the good work and enjoy the healthy new you.

A FINAL WORD ABOUT NICOTINE REPLACEMENT PRODUCTS

If you're using the patch, gum, or other nicotine replacement products, you're probably using them less frequently and may have stopped using them altogether. Some advice may be important here. First, remember that the nicotine in these products is not enough to be dangerous and that you want to make sure you really don't need it any longer before you give it up. So, if you are still feeling some urges, you may want to continue your nicotine replacement regimen, perhaps at a lower strength and/or dosage. Second, even though you may feel confident that you've quit smoking for good and no longer need to use nicotine replacement, you may want to keep some patches or gum handy to help deal with unanticipated urges. If you continue to use nicotine replacement products for more than 6 months please be sure to use them with your doctor's approval.

Staying Smoke-free for Good

You made it through the toughest parts of quitting smoking and stuck with it. For this, you should be very proud of yourself and what you've accomplished. But that doesn't mean that your efforts should stop. You will still need to be on guard against roadblocks. Remember, anticipating temptations or roadblocks goes a long way to overcoming them. The following is a list of some of the strategies you learned in this book for staying smoke-free. Use it if you are trying to prepare for a tough roadblock, want a quick refresher, or need some positive reinforcement. We've included page numbers for more detailed information on each topic if you would like to review the material more closely. Use the blank spaces at the end of the list to fill in temptations or roadblocks you need to watch for and any strategies you may have discovered on your own. Maybe you'll want to highlight the ones that have been particularly useful to you.

Summing it Up: Staying Smoke-free

- You made a list of your reasons to quit smoking and put it in your purse or wallet to remind you of why staying smoke-free was and is important to you when the urge to smoke arises (page 61).

- You asked your family and friends for support and encouragement. You asked one of them to be your quitting coach and to work with you more closely, especially for when you need extra help or support (page 64).

- You monitored your smoking patterns and learned how to anticipate the situations that would be most tempting to you or pose the biggest roadblocks to staying off cigarettes (page 69).

- You learned how to use relaxation exercises to cope with the stress or nervousness associated with quitting (page 72).

- You learned how to make healthy snack choices to fight cravings to smoke (page 84).

- You learned how to use physical activity to distract yourself from the urge to smoke and to replace your smoking habit with healthier ones (page 109).

- You practiced using positive self-talk to reinforce your resolve to quit (page 148).

- You practiced saying no while keeping communication assertive and upbeat (page 152).

- You learned how to prepare for social situations in which people may be smoking (pages 154–158).

- Other strategies I discovered:

_____

_____

_____

_____

_____

_____

_____

_____

ACTION ITEM

WHAT WORKED BEST FOR ME

Take a minute to review the list of lessons and strategies you learned in this book and any new ones you discovered. Write down the ones that worked best for you in the spaces below.

1. **Example:** Having my reasons for quitting handy really kept me from lapsing back into smoking.

2. **Example:** Replacing my smoking with other habits, such as having a piece of fruit to combat the urge to smoke, was a great way to start building more healthy routines overall.

3.

4.

5.

6.

7.

ACTION ITEM

REMAINING "HOT SPOTS"

Now take another few minutes to review the temptations and roadblocks that have been most troublesome to you. Which ones do you still need to watch out for? Are there upcoming events (a major challenge at work, an anniversary of a sad event in your life, a son or daughter getting married) that may pose problems for you? Think about these and figure out what you will need to be careful with and how you can cope with them.

Here's an example:

Hot Spot: Celebrations like weddings, New Year's Eve, Christmas day, my birthday.

Danger Signs: Thinking about how much fun it will be to just cut loose and enjoy myself for a day or so.

Strategy:
1. Before such celebrations, think about all my blessings and remind myself that not smoking is one of my blessings and that remaining a nonsmoker will give me more to look forward to.
2. Figure out some other ways to "cut loose" that won't put me at risk for smoking.
3. Work out some specific plans for how to avoid parts of the celebrations that may really tempt me.

Hot Spot:

Danger Signs:

Strategy:

Hot Spot:

Danger Signs:

Strategy:

Hot Spot:

Danger Signs:

Strategy:

Hot Spot:

Danger Signs:

Strategy:

Review these Hot Spots and your plans for coping with them every week or so over the next few months.

Physical Activity, Healthy Eating, and the Healthy New You

"Quitting smoking got me thinking about all my not-so-healthy routines, especially my high-fat eating habits and lack of exercise. When I quit, I started to work on my weight. It really gave me a new lease on life. Now I feel much more energetic and good about myself." (Toni, age 72)

Physical Activity for the New You

Now that you've been smoke-free for a while, have you found that being active got a little easier? Do you have more energy to get through the day? Have your walks gotten more brisk or perhaps even turned into a jog? If you haven't been working on it, these are the kinds of things that you can look forward to once you get started and stay with it for a while. Why not go back to chapter five and give it a try this time? Beginning is half of every action and, as Toni's story shows, beginning physical activity is a big step toward a happier and healthier life.

In the last seven chapters, you've learned a lot about physical activity. Let's review some of the things we've covered. If you haven't been active, take a look at the list of topics we covered; it might motivate you to get started. If you have been working on physical activity, remind yourself of the things you learned and try some new ideas to intensify and/or add to what you are already doing.

The following is a list of some strategies you learned for how to get more active and how to use physical activity to help you stay smoke-free. We've included page numbers for more detailed information on each topic if you would like to review the material more closely. Use the blank spaces at the end of the list to fill in any strategies you discovered on your own, or maybe you'll want to highlight the ones that have been particularly useful to you.

- You learned that even small bouts of physical activity can add up (pages 41–45).

- You reminded yourself of all the benefits of physical activity: reducing stress and building up your energy, lowering your risk for serious diseases, and how physical activity can help you manage your weight and improve your self-image and confidence (pages 44–45).

- You identified people who can help and encourage you to quit smoking and get more active (page 96).

- You identified roadblocks that might get in the way of your becoming more active and made a plan for getting past them (page 101).

- You set some basic goals for getting more active and planned for how you were going to achieve them (pages 103–105).

- You made a time study of your daily routines to see how active you were and to locate opportunities for fitting physical activity into your day (pages 98–99).

- You made a daily physical activity schedule. You learned some tips for how to intensify your routine and make it more interesting, such as trying to be active at different times of the day, combining shorter bouts of physical activity into longer ones, and finding a form of exercise you really enjoy (pages 138–139).

• Other strategies I discovered:

_____

_____

_____

_____

_____

_____

_____

_____

Now let's focus on what worked best for you. Think about the tips you learned and the Action Items you completed. Make a list of the strategies that worked best for you. This list may include activities that helped you to get started, those that you used to quit smoking, and those that have become a part of your routine.

Physical Activity Can Be Fun

In the last chapter, you started to make physical activity more a part of your routine. Now that you have started to build a schedule for physical activity, let's make sure that you're on the right track and having fun. Physical activity does not have to be a hassle. On the contrary, it can add new dimensions to your

ACTION ITEM: *Physical Activity*

WHAT WORKED BEST FOR ME

Take a minute to review the list of lessons and strategies you learned in this book and any new ones you discovered. Write down the ones that worked best for you in the spaces below.

1.**Example:** Taking 2-minute walks when the urges came helped a lot. Now I walk all the time.

2.**Example:** Having a friend to be active with me was key. My racquetball partner really helped keep me motivated.

3.

4.

5.

6.

7.

life—new friends, new hobbies, new outlook, new body—that can be fun and rewarding. And like Toni, you may even surprise yourself and do things you didn't think you could do.

Having a positive outlook and enjoying the activities you do will help you stick with them over the long run. But feeling frustrated about exercise can throw you off course. If you are still working out your routine, let's find ways to get it right and make physical activity something you enjoy and look forward to. Check in with yourself every month or two, and ask yourself the following questions. This will help you to get in touch with how you feel about your physical activity routine and let you know whether it's time for a change.

- *Do I enjoy physical activity?*
  If you find that you are enjoying your physical activity routine, then it seems you have found the right set of activities for you. Keep up the good work, and remember to check in with yourself from time to time. Even if you are happy with what you are doing, it can't hurt to experiment with new things and liven up your routine a little.

- *Am I bored, frustrated, or distracted when I exercise?*
  If you find that you are bored, frustrated, or distracted, a little trial and error can help. There will always be distractions, but if you aren't enjoying the activities you are doing, try to experiment with them until you get it right. You might try fitting your activity in at a different time of day when you aren't so rushed or distracted by other things. Or you might try doing a different activity, but keeping the same time slot you already set aside. Again, classes are great for adding variety to your routine.

- *Do I feel good physically when I am active?*
  If your answer to this question is no, make sure that you are not doing too much. You may be straining some muscles.

Stretch before doing any physical activity and take it slow. A gradual approach can take away some of the frustration of feeling that your body is not keeping up with what your mind wants it to do. Refer back to page 104 in chapter five for some tips about stretching and how to get active safely and gradually, and make sure to check with your physician if you experience persistent physical discomfort as a result of your physical activity. With the money you will be saving from not smoking, you may also consider trying a couple of sessions with a personal trainer. Trainers are available at most gyms and YMCAs and some of them even offer free consultations as part of your orientation. By measuring your level of endurance, a trainer can work with you to create an activity plan that is safe and effective. A trainer can also help you decide when to increase your level of physical activity and are often great for keeping you motivated. Trainers are also helpful for making decisions about adding a strength training program into your routine.

- *Do I feel a sense of accomplishment from my physical activity?* We hope so. You've done some really great work. Quitting smoking is a difficult thing to do and you managed to do it and work on getting more active. These are two of the main ingredients in building a healthy new you, and you are well on your way. If you aren't feeling good about what you've accomplished, remind yourself of all that you've learned and how much time you've spent working on your health. Practice a little positive self-talk to build your confidence and get back on track. You quit smoking! This is a major accomplishment.

Finally, if you find that for some reason you get entirely thrown off track, go back to chapter five and use what you've learned to get back into the habit of being physically active, even if it means starting over. There are many things in life that can

ACTION ITEM

ACTIVITY GOALS FOR YOUR FUTURE

Write down some basic activity goals for the months and years ahead. You may be doing a couple of 15-minute walks a week but want to increase it or take them more regularly. Maybe you're more active than that, but work deadlines seem to get in the way of your sticking to your routine. Think about what you want to accomplish in the future, what could get in the way, and some strategies for overcoming the roadblocks to your reaching your goals. Below are some sentences to complete and help you think about your activity goals:

Example:

In the coming year, I **want** to: *be more physically active by taking 30-minute walks for five days of every week.*

In the coming year, I **don't** want to: *let work deadlines and stress get in the way of taking those 30-minute walks.*

In the coming year, I always want to remember that, **when** *I get very busy or stressed at work,* **I need to** *plan my schedule and fit exercise into my day even it means doing two 15-minute walks, instead of doing it all at once.*

In the coming year, I **want** to: _____

In the coming year, I **don't** want to: _____

In the coming year, I always want to
remember that, **when:** _____
I need to: _____

get in the way of one's routine: holidays, vacations, being extra busy, sickness, pregnancy. If possible, try to plan ahead. But if you cannot, try starting up your physical activity again when things calm down. Remember those benefits, and be confident about how much you've learned and already accomplished.

Healthy Eating for the New You

Healthy eating is a part of the overall picture of your health, just as being smoke-free and physically active are. You may have used healthy snack choices to help you with your smoking and to satisfy your cravings. Or maybe you started to work on having a more balanced eating style overall. If so, keep up the good work—it'll help you stay smoke-free and manage your weight over the long run. If you haven't been thinking much about your eating habits, you may want to start now. Doing so can boost your energy level and self-confidence, help you manage and eventually lose weight, and reduce your risk of serious diseases such as coronary heart disease, cancer, diabetes, and others.

The following is a list of some of the strategies you learned for making healthy eating choices and staying smoke-free. We've included page numbers for more detailed information on each topic if you would like to review the material more closely. Use the blank spaces at the end of the list to fill in any strategies you discovered on your own. Maybe you'll want to highlight the ones that have been particularly useful to you.

Summing It Up: Making Healthy Eating Choices

- You identified people who could encourage and support you and your eating choices (pages 116–117).

- You studied when, where, and how you eat by keeping a

ACTION ITEM: *Eating*

WHAT WORKED BEST FOR ME

Take a minute to review the list of lessons and strategies you learned in this book and any new ones you discovered. Write down the ones that worked best for you in the spaces below.

1.**Example:** I started drinking water with my food. It helps me to eat what I need instead of eating too much.

2.**Example:** I keep a fruit bowl on the table and now I eat much more fruit because it's so easy to get to.

3.

4.

5.

6.

7.

food diary. You thought more closely about what you ate, including the kinds of foods, how much, and how you felt when you ate them. You found ways to make your meals more healthy and nutritious (pages 118–120).

◆ You learned how to slow yourself down when eating and how to make healthier foods more readily available to you (page 124).

◆ You learned tips for how to eat healthier snacks and to choose healthier alternatives to your regular eating habits (pages 128–129).

◆ You identified roadblocks, such as time constraints and cravings, that might have gotten in the way of your success at staying smoke-free and making healthy eating choices and you planned for how you were going to get past them (pages 122–123).

◆ You started to think about having a more balanced eating style (pages 130–131).

Keeping Up the Good Work

At the beginning of this chapter, we asked you how it felt to be a nonsmoker. We bet it feels great. You've done some excellent work here, and hope that you are celebrating your success and feeling confident with your efforts to have a longer and healthier life. You should never let your guard down completely, but you'll know you have made it as a nonsmoker when:

◆ Your urges are few and far between.

◆ You realize you've been through one of your former roadblock situations and didn't even think about smoking.

ACTION ITEM

HEALTHY EATING GOALS FOR YOUR FUTURE

Write down some basic goals for healthy eating over the upcoming months. You may have improved your snacking behaviors by eating healthier foods between meals, but want to add more fruits and vegetables to your diet. Or maybe you've changed some of your personal relationships that have made healthy eating difficult for you but want to work on eating healthier when you are dining out. Think about what you want to accomplish in the future, what could get in the way, and some strategies for overcoming roadblocks. Below are some sentences to complete to help you think about your healthy eating goals:

Example

In the coming year, I **want** to: *make healthier eating choices when I am eating out with certain friends or family members.*

In the coming year, I **don't** want to: *lapse out of my healthy eating habits when I am eating out with certain friends or family members.*

In the coming year, I always want to remember that, **when** *I am eating out,* **I need to** *choose a restaurant that offers healthy food options and make sure to remind my friends and family that I am trying to make healthy food choices and not cave in when we are together.*

In the coming year, I **want** to: _____

In the coming year, I **don't** want to: _____

In the coming year, I always want to
remember that, **when:** _____
I need to: _____

ACTION ITEM

LONG-TERM GOALS AND HOW QUITTING WILL POSITIVELY AFFECT MY FUTURE

Make a list of some long-term goals or things you're looking forward to in the upcoming years and how quitting smoking has changed your life for the better.

Example 1

- In the next few years, I am looking forward to: getting a promotion at work, having a healthy, energetic lifestyle, and saving money for my child's college fund.

- Being smoke-free will help me: keep my energy up and stay on my toes at work, and help me to stay physically active and trim, and save the money I used to spend on cigarettes.

- In the next few years, I am looking forward to: _____

- Being smoke-free will help me: _____
_____

- In the next few years, I am looking forward to: _____

- Being smoke-free will help me: _____
_____

- In the next few years, I am looking forward to: _____

- Being smoke-free will help me: _____
_____

◆ You enjoy not smoking.

◆ You don't have feelings of nostalgia about smoking.

◆ You wish you could reach out to people who still smoke and help them quit.

◆ You realize you sometimes have thoughts like "This used to be a time when I'd smoke," or "A cigarette might be nice right now," but you no longer have uncontrollable urges that push you to want to smoke.

◆ You really understand that it's easier to have none than one.

Another way to reinforce your resolve to stay smoke-free is to think about what giving up cigarettes has meant to your life and the good times and opportunities you will have now that cigarettes are no longer a part of it. The Action Item on page 179 can help you do just that. Maybe you are just trying to take it one day at a time. But why not try looking for how giving up smoking will mean a better life for you and for your loved ones?

Finally, we want to wish you the best of luck in achieving the goals you set for yourself. We hope this book has given you some tools that will help you achieve these and any new goals you set for yourself in the future. Staying smoke-free, being active, and having a healthy eating style are the foundation of a long and healthy life, and you've made significant progress in each of these areas. Keep up the good work and enjoy your success. And once again, congratulations!

Sample Menus
and Recipes for
Healthy Eating

9

Now that you've learned how to manage your weight by making healthier eating choices and becoming more physically active, we can tie in some of the lessons you learned in previous chapters about making healthy eating choices with easy-to-follow daily menus. Most of the meals can be made with the ingredients already in your cupboard, and won't take much time to prepare. Menus for breakfast, lunch and dinner—as well as in-between snacks for when you might crave a cigarette or need something to tide you over to the next meal—are included. There is also a listing of recipes, each with detailed nutritional information by serving amount. For the recipes, be sure to eat only one serving of each item. For example, if the menu calls for a Strawberry Yogurt Shake, be sure to remember that the recipe is for two servings. You can decide to save one serving for later, or halve the ingredient portions in the recipe. General information about serving sizes is available in chapter two (pages 48–49).

The menus in this chapter also include suggestions for low-calorie beverages to accompany your meals. Monitoring your beverage intake is an important part of watching your weight because the calories in beverages can add up if you are not careful. Below are some tasty low- and no-calorie options that can help you to keep your calorie count to a minimum. And, of course, drinking water at any time of the day can fill you up and is an absolute must for good health.

- Iced tea (if unsweetened, add some Sweet 'N Low or Equal for the low-calorie option)

- Flavored waters

- Diet sodas

- Fat-free or 1% milk

- Water (we recommend 8–10 glasses of water per day)

Note: These beverages can be consumed liberally, although you may want to watch how much diet soda you drink if it contains caffeine. See the sidebar below on caffeine.

A WORD ABOUT CAFFEINE

As you continue to work on staying smoke-free, you're likely to feel the effects of the caffeine a little more than when you were smoking. We suggest that you try decreasing the amount of caffeine you consume. You don't have to stop eating or drinking caffeinated products completely, but cutting back can really help improve your health. One way to cut down on your caffeine intake is to try making a "half-n-half" cup of coffee. A "half-n-half" cup is a mixture of half-caffeinated, half-decaffeinated coffee. Another way to cut down is to choose decaffeinated versions of your favorite beverages. For example, try replacing your morning or mid-afternoon coffee with an herbal tea. Or, drink decaffeinated sodas or low-calorie flavored ice teas, which are available in most grocery stores and soda machines.

Menu 1

BREAKFAST

- $^1/_2$ cup oatmeal with cinnamon, honey and raisins, fresh apple slices, or applesauce
- 1 cup plain low-fat yogurt with your favorite fruits, such as strawberries, blueberries, and/or bananas
- Coffee or herbal tea (with fat-free or 1% milk and/or sugar substitute)

LUNCH

- Turkey Sandwich
  2 slices light whole-wheat bread
  2 oz fresh roasted turkey or 2 slices turkey lunch meat
  Romaine lettuce and slice of tomato
  As desired: honey mustard (if you want to use mayonnaise, be sure to read the nutrition facts on the label to see how much fat it contains. Low-calorie mayonnaise is available in most stores.)
- Carrot Raisin Salad (see recipe on page 192)

MID-AFTERNOON SNACK

- Part-skim mozzarella cheese stick

DINNER

- Fish-n-Chips
  Fish Fillets (see recipe on page 205)
  and Fantastic Fries (see recipe on page 204)

DESSERT

- Pistachio Surprise
  Mix one package of instant pistachio pudding mix, 1 can (16 oz) crushed pineapple and two small containers of low-fat plain yogurt together and refrigerate until ready to serve.

LATE-NIGHT SNACK

- Glass of fat-free or 1% milk with cocoa

Menu 2

BREAKFAST
- Strawberry Yogurt Shake (see recipe on page 190)
- 1 cup cold cereal with fat-free or 1% milk
- Coffee or herbal tea (with fat-free or 1% milk and/or sugar substitute)

LUNCH
- Super Spinach Salad (see recipe on page 203)
- Spice-n-Rice (see recipe on page 200)

MID-AFTERNOON SNACK
- Rice cakes with apple butter (see recipe for apple butter on page 191)

DINNER
- Crispy Coated Chicken (see recipe on page 195)
- Steamed carrots, string beans, and onions. After steaming, add one teaspoon olive oil and pinch of salt and pepper to taste.

DESSERT
- Gelatin with fruit. Try making parfait style with a layer of gelatin, a layer of fruit, and a layer of low-fat whipped topping.

LATE-NIGHT SNACK
- Frozen Pops: freeze in paper cups with a wooden stick, any of the following: applesauce, crushed pineapple, or fruit juices.

Menu 3

BREAKFAST

- Apple butter on toast (see recipe for apple butter on page 191)
- 1 cup cold cereal with fat-free or 1% milk
- Coffee or herbal tea (with fat-free or 1% milk and/or sugar substitute)

LUNCH

- Tuna Sandwich
  Mix tuna (if from can, buy tuna packed in water instead of oil) with one teaspoon light mayonnaise and one teaspoon of relish. Spread onto two pieces of whole-wheat toast and add spinach, lettuce, or any other leafy green vegetable and some onion or tomato if you wish.
- One piece of fruit, or if you crave something crunchy, have some pretzels or low-fat baked chips.

MID-AFTERNOON SNACK

- Air-popped or low-fat popcorn

DINNER

- Vegetable Burritos (see recipe on page 196)
- White or yellow rice

DESSERT

- Apple Raisin Toast—Toast one slice of raisin bread. Microwave sliced apples with cinnamon on top. Put the apples on the toast. Add light whipped topping if you wish.

LATE-NIGHT SNACK

- Fresh vegetables such as carrots, celery, cauliflower, and peppers

Menu 4

BREAKFAST

- Fruit Parfait
  Cut up some fresh fruit and put some low-fat plain or
  vanilla yogurt on top. Add a layer of granola-like cereal.
  Then add another layer of fruit and yogurt. Add a dash
  of cinnamon or nutmeg on top.
- Coffee or herbal tea (with fat-free or 1% milk and/or sugar
  substitute)

LUNCH

- Homemade soup – Caraway Cabbage or Northeast Cream-that-
  Broccoli soup (see recipes on pages 193 and 198 respectively)
- Whole-wheat crackers or saltines
- Garden side salad with chopped vegetables of choice and light
  dressing (one tablespoon extra virgin olive oil, tablespoon of
  balsamic vinaigrette and fresh ground pepper, add oregano for
  taste). If you are in a rush, grab a salad at your local fast food
  restaurant, and choose the low-fat dressing option.

MID-AFTERNOON SNACK

- Peaches, plums, pineapple (fresh or canned), pears, and/or berries,
  such as blueberries, raspberries, or strawberries. Try freezing the
  berries before eating.

DINNER

- Chicken-Cabbage Stir-Fry (see recipe on page 199)
- Steamed white rice, with broth/seasoning from the stir-fry
- Serve with Garden side salad

DESSERT

- Banana slice: freeze a very ripe banana half on a stick, dip in low-
  fat yogurt and sprinkle with wheat germ or high-fiber cereal.

LATE-NIGHT SNACK

- Crushed graham crackers mixed into low-fat yogurt.

Menu 5

BREAKFAST

- Poached egg spread over slice of whole-wheat toast. Add $1/2$ cup of spinach placed between egg and toast and some fresh ground pepper on top, if desired.
- Coffee or herbal tea (with fat-free or 1% milk and/or sugar substitute)

LUNCH

- Cagey Midwest Corn and Black Bean Chili (see recipe on page 194)
- Homemade Tortilla Chips (see recipe on page 202)

MID-AFTERNOON SNACK

- Cut-up vegetables with low-fat ranch dressing

DINNER

- Chicken and Rice (see recipe on page 201)
- Ranch Style Vegetables (see recipe on page 197)

DESSERT

- Peach, Lemon or Mandarin Orange Ripieno
  Hollow out a peach, lemon, or mandarin orange and
  fill with sorbet of the same flavor.

LATE-NIGHT SNACK

- 2 graham crackers, or 5 wheat crackers with
  two tablespoons of low-fat cottage cheese

RECIPES

Strawberry Yogurt Shake *(serves 2)*

INGREDIENTS:

$\frac{1}{2}$ cup pineapple juice
$1\frac{1}{2}$ cups frozen, unsweetened strawberries
$\frac{3}{4}$ cup plain low-fat yogurt
1 teaspoon sugar

TO PREPARE:

1. Add ingredients, in order listed above, to blender container.
2. Cover blender container with lid.
3. Blend at medium speed, until thick and smooth.
4. Serve immediately.

NUTRITIONAL INFORMATION *(per serving)*:
Calories, 146; carbohydrate, 27 g; protein, 5 g;
fat, 2 g; saturated fat, 0 g; cholesterol, 6 mg; fiber, 3 g;
sodium, 63 mg.

Apple Butter *(serves 6)*

INGREDIENTS:

6 apples, cored and sliced
$\frac{1}{2}$ cup unsweetened apple juice
$\frac{1}{2}$ cup water
cinnamon or cloves to taste

TO PREPARE:

1. In a medium saucepan, simmer apples in apple juice and water until they are soft.
2. Remove contents from pan and place into blender container.
3. Cover blender container with lid and blend until smooth.
4. Add cinnamon or cloves to taste.
5. Return mixture to saucepan and cook slowly for another 30 minutes.
6. Use as a spread for bread or toast or serve with plain low-fat yogurt.

NUTRITIONAL INFORMATION *(per serving)*:

Calories, 36; carbohydrate, 9 g; protein, 0 g; fat, 0 g; saturated fat, 0 g; fiber 1 g; sodium, 0 mg.

Carrot Raisin Salad *(serves 4)*

INGREDIENTS:

4 medium carrots, peeled and grated
¼ cup of raisins
2 teaspoons sugar
juice of 1 lemon

TO PREPARE:

1. In a medium bowl, thoroughly mix carrots, raisins, sugar, and lemon juice.
2. Serve chilled.

NUTRITIONAL INFORMATION *(per serving)*:
Calories, 68; carbohydrate, 16 g; protein, 1 g; fat, 0 g; saturated fat, 0 g; fiber, 5 g; sodium, 36 mg.

Caraway Cabbage Soup *(serves 4)*

INGREDIENTS:

1 teaspoon vegetable oil
1 cup chopped onions
1 russet potato, peeled and cut into $^1/_2$-inch cubes
4 cups chopped cabbage
1 teaspoon caraway seeds
4 cups low-sodium vegetable or chicken broth
$^1/_4$ teaspoon salt
$^1/_4$ teaspoon pepper

TO PREPARE:

1. Heat the oil in a large saucepan on medium heat.
2. Cook onion until it begins to wilt (about 2 minutes).
3. Add potatoes, cabbage, and caraway seeds and stir-fry 1 minute.
4. Pour in broth and season with salt and pepper.
5. Bring to a boil, reduce heat, and simmer 1 hour.
6. Serve with a piece of crusty rye bread.

NUTRITIONAL INFORMATION *(per serving)*:
Calories, 102; carbohydrate, 19 g; protein, 2 g; fat, 2 g; saturated fat, 0 g; fiber, 3 g; sodium, 222 mg.

Cagey Midwest Corn and Black Bean Chili *(serves 6-8)*

INGREDIENTS:

1 yellow onion, sliced
1 teaspoon vegetable oil
1 red bell pepper, diced
1 green bell pepper, diced
1–2 tablespoons chopped, canned jalapeño peppers
3 tablespoons minced garlic
1 pound frozen corn
1½ cups cooked black beans or 1 15-ounce can black
    beans, rinsed and drained
1 28-ounce can peeled, diced tomatoes
2 packets chili seasoning or chili powder to taste
3 cups low sodium beef broth
hot sauce to taste
pepper to taste (optional)
1 cup fat-free sour cream (optional)
½ cup fat-free cheddar cheese (optional), chopped green
    onion, or cilantro (optional)

TO PREPARE:

1. Sauté onion in vegetable oil for 8 minutes on medium-high heat.
2. Add bell peppers, jalapeño, and garlic and sauté for
   4–5 minutes more, taking care not to burn garlic.
3. Add the next five ingredients and stir well.
4. Bring pot to a boil, then reduce heat and simmer
   for at least 30 minutes.
5. Add hot sauce and pepper to taste.
6. Top with sour cream, cheese, green onion,
   and/or cilantro if desired, and serve.

NUTRITIONAL INFORMATION *(per serving)*:

*Calories, 162; carbohydrate, 27 g; protein, 9 g; fat, 2 g;
saturated fat, 0 g; fiber, 6 g; sodium, 107 mg.*

Crispy Coated Chicken *(serves 6)*

INGREDIENTS:

1 cup fat-free milk
1 egg
1 cup all-purpose flour
pepper to taste
$\frac{1}{2}$ teaspoon garlic powder or oregano (optional)
2 cups crushed cornflakes cereal
3 pounds skinless chicken pieces, rinsed and dried
non-stick cooking spray

TO PREPARE:

1. Preheat oven to 350°F.
2. In small bowl, mix together milk and egg with flour, pepper, and garlic powder or oregano.
3. Put crushed cornflakes in shallow pan.
4. Dip chicken into batter then roll into crushed cornflakes.
5. Lightly spray shallow baking pan with non-stick cooking spray.
6. Lightly spray chicken with non-stick cooking spray.
7. Bake at 350°F for 1 hour, or until chicken is done.
8. Serve warm.

NUTRITIONAL INFORMATION *(per serving)*:
Calories, 573; carbohydrate, 46 g; protein, 77 g;
fat, 9 g; saturated fat, 3 g; cholesterol, 229 mg; fiber, 2 g;
sodium, 433 mg.

Vegetable Burritos

INGREDIENTS:

1 teaspoon vegetable oil
2 cups onion
3 cloves garlic
1 cup red bell pepper
2 cups sliced mushrooms
1 teaspoon chili powder
dash of salt
$1/2$ teaspoon cumin (optional)
$1^1/2$ cups cooked black beans or 1 15-ounce can black
   beans, rinsed and drained
4 flour tortillas
$1/2$ cup chopped cilantro (optional)

TO PREPARE:

1. Preheat oven to 350°F.
2. Heat vegetable oil in a high-sided skillet.
3. Cook onions until soft and slightly golden, about 5 minutes.
4. Add garlic, bell pepper, mushrooms, chili powder, salt, and cumin. Cook until vegetables are tender, about 5 minutes.
5. Stir in black beans and heat through.
6. Heat tortillas in a paper bag in microwave, about 1 minute.
7. Lay warm tortillas on counter. Divide the filling among them and scatter cilantro on top.
8. Roll into a neat package, turning in the sides.
9. Lay in a baking dish covered lightly with aluminum foil and warm through in the oven, 10 minutes.
10. Serve warm.

NUTRITIONAL INFORMATION *(per serving)*:
Calories, 233; carbohydrate, 44 g; protein, 3 g; fat, 5 g; saturated fat, 1 g; fiber, 9 g; sodium, 362 mg.

Ranch-Style Vegetables *(serves 4)*

INGREDIENTS:

1 cup cauliflower, broken into bite-sized pieces
2 cups broccoli, broken into bite-sized pieces
$3/4$ cup sliced carrots
$1/2$ cup sliced celery
$1/2$ cup chopped onion
$1/4$ teaspoon dried dill weed
$1 1/2$ tablespoons lemon juice
2 tablespoons fat-free or reduced-fat ranch-style dressing

TO PREPARE:

1. Fill a $1 1/2$-quart microwave-safe dish with vegetables.
2. Add dill and lemon juice.
3. Cover and microwave 5 to 8 minutes.
4. Drain and mix in dressing.
5. Serve warm.

NUTRITIONAL INFORMATION *(per serving)*:

Calories, 70; carbohydrate, 11 g; protein, 2 g; fat, 0 g; saturated fat, 0 g; fiber, 3 g; sodium, 112 mg.

Northeast Cream-that-Broccoli Soup (serves 6-8)

INGREDIENTS:

3 medium brown russet potatoes
1½ pounds fresh broccoli
5 cloves garlic
1 teaspoon vegetable oil
3½ cups fat-free, low sodium chicken broth
salt to taste
pepper to taste (optional)
½ cup grated Parmesan cheese for garnish (optional)

TO PREPARE:

1. Bring a large pot of water to a boil.
2. Cut potatoes into quarters, leaving skin on. Add to pot of boiling water.
3. Cook for 20 to 25 minutes, until potatoes are very soft.
4. Remove any tough ends from the broccoli.
5. Chop broccoli into bite-sized pieces. Steam for 5 to 7 minutes, using a steamer insert that fits into larger pot.
6. Peel and mince garlic. Heat oil in small pan on medium heat.
7. Gently sauté garlic for 3 to 4 minutes, until soft and light brown.
8. Drain potatoes.
9. Blend potatoes, broccoli, and garlic with chicken broth in a blender. Work in batches since the blender will not be large enough for all ingredients at the same time.
10. Pour puree into a large pot and reheat. Add salt and pepper.
11. Serve warm. Garnish with Parmesan cheese.

NUTRITIONAL INFORMATION *(per serving)*:
Calories, 185; carbohydrate, 25 g; protein, 10 g; fat, 5 g; saturated fat, 2 g; fiber, 5 g; sodium, 394 g.

Chicken-Cabbage Stir-Fry *(serves 4)*

INGREDIENTS:

3 chicken breast halves, skinned and boned
1 teaspoon oil
3 cups green cabbage, cut in $\frac{1}{2}$-inch slices
1 tablespoon cornstarch
$\frac{1}{4}$ teaspoon garlic powder
$\frac{1}{2}$ teaspoon ground ginger
$\frac{1}{2}$ cup water
1 tablespoon soy sauce

TO PREPARE:

1. Cut chicken breast halves into strips.
2. Heat oil in frying pan.
3. Add chicken strips and stir fry over moderately high heat, turning pieces constantly, until lightly browned (about 2 to 3 minutes).
4. Add cabbage; stir fry 2 minutes until cabbage is tender-crisp.
5. Mix cornstarch and seasonings; add to water and soy sauce, mixing until smooth.
6. Stir into chicken mixture.
7. Cook until thickened and pieces are coated, about 1 minute.

NUTRITIONAL INFORMATION *(per serving)*:
Calories, 146; carbohydrate, 5 g; protein, 27 g; fat, 2 g; saturated fat, 0 g; cholesterol, 50 mg; fiber, 1 g; sodium, 325 mg.

Spice-n-Rice *(serves 8)*

INGREDIENTS:

non-stick cooking spray
$1/2$ cup chopped onion
$1/2$ cup chopped sweet red pepper
$2^1/2$ cups water
1 teaspoon chicken-flavored bouillon
$1/2$ teaspoon ground cumin
$1/8$ teaspoon hot sauce
1 cup rice, uncooked

TO PREPARE:

1. Coat a medium saucepan with non-stick cooking spray and place over medium heat until hot.
2. Add onion and pepper, sauté 5 minutes or until tender.
3. Add water, bouillon, cumin, and hot sauce and bring to a boil.
4. Stir in rice, cover, and reduce heat. Simmer until rice is tender and liquid is absorbed (about 20 minutes).

NUTRITIONAL INFORMATION *(per serving)*:
Calories, 90; carbohydrate, 20 g; protein, 2 g;
fat, 0 g; saturated fat, 0 g; cholesterol, 0 mg; fiber, 4 g;
sodium, 50 mg.

Chicken and Rice *(serves 6)*

INGREDIENTS:

1 tablespoon olive or canola oil
6 small pieces of skinless chicken breast
1 large onion, diced
3 minced garlic cloves
1 chopped green bell pepper
1¼ cups chopped tomatoes
½ teaspoon salt
¼ teaspoon ground black pepper
¼ teaspoon cilantro
1 bay leaf
½ teaspoon paprika
2 cups water
1½ cups white wine
10 ounces frozen green peas
2 cups long-grain white rice, uncooked

TO PREPARE:

1. In a large non-stick skillet, heat oil over medium heat.
2. Sauté chicken breasts until lightly browned on all sides, then set chicken aside on paper towels.
3. In skillet, add onion, garlic, and green pepper, and sauté 3 to 5 minutes.
4. Add tomatoes, salt, black pepper, cilantro, bay leaf, paprika, and water. Cover and bring to a boil.
5. Add the chicken and simmer over medium-low heat for 30 minutes.
6. Add the wine, peas, and rice and simmer for 20 minutes more.

NUTRITIONAL INFORMATION *(per serving)*:
Calories, 430; carbohydrate, 66 g; protein, 32 g; fat, 4 g; saturated fat, .5 g; cholesterol, 35 mg; fiber, 4 g; sodium, 350 mg.

Homemade Tortilla Chips *(makes 8 cups)*

INGREDIENTS:
12 thin corn tortillas
water
salt
non-stick cooking spray

TO PREPARE:
1. Put each tortilla in water and drain.
2. Lay each one flat and sprinkle with salt.
3. Stack the tortillas and cut into 8 pieces.
4. Spray baking sheet with non-stick spray and arrange tortilla slices in a single layer.
5. Bake in a 500°F for 4 minutes, then turn with tongs and continue baking until crisp and brown (about 2 more minutes).
6. Repeat until all chips are cooked.

NUTRITIONAL INFORMATION *(per serving)*:
Calories, 110; carbohydrate, 22 g; protein, 2 g; fat, 3.5g; saturated fat, 0 g; cholesterol, 0 mg; fiber, 4 g; sodium, 0 mg.

Super Spinach Salad *(serves 8-12)*

INGREDIENTS:

4 cups torn lettuce or other salad greens
4 cups fresh spinach torn in bite-size pieces
1 fresh, sliced or 1 can (11 ounces) mandarin
    orange sections, drained
1 cup sliced fresh mushrooms
1 small onion, sliced and separated into rings
$1/2$ cup low-calorie Italian dressing

TO PREPARE:

1. Combine all ingredients except dressing in a large bowl.
2. Keep refrigerated until serving time.
3. Toss with dressing.

NUTRITIONAL INFORMATION *(per serving)*:

Calories, 35; carbohydrate, 7 g; protein, 1 g; fat, 1 g;
saturated fat, 0 g; cholesterol, 0 mg; fiber, 2 g;
sodium, 95 mg.

Fantastic Fries *(serves 4)*

INGREDIENTS:

4 medium-sized potatoes
4 teaspoons olive or canola oil
non-stick cooking spray
garlic powder
onion powder
salt

TO PREPARE:

1. Preheat oven to 400°F.
2. Cut potatoes into long french fry shapes.
3. Keep potatoes in bowl of cold water until you are finished cutting.
4. Drain water, then add oil and toss until the uncooked fries are coated.
5. Spray a large baking sheet with non-stick cooking spray and spread out potatoes.
6. Sprinkle with garlic and onion powder, and salt to taste.
7. Bake for about 20 minutes, then remove from the oven, turn over and bake for another 10–20 minutes or until crisp.

NUTRITIONAL INFORMATION *(per serving)*:
Calories, 200; carbohydrate, 37 g; protein, 4 g; fat, 5 g; saturated fat, 1 g; cholesterol, 0 mg; fiber, 4 g; sodium, 90 mg.

Fish Fillets *(serves 4)*

INGREDIENTS:

non-stick cooking spray
2 tablespoons plain non-fat yogurt
1 tablespoon olive or canola oil
1$\frac{1}{2}$ teaspoons lemon juice
4 tablespoons bread crumbs
1 pound fresh (or frozen, but thawed) flounder
    or sole fillets
1 teaspoon sea salt
$\frac{1}{2}$ teaspoon paprika

TO PREPARE:

1. Preheat oven to 475°F.
2. Spray baking pan with plenty of cooking spray.
3. Mix yogurt, oil, and juice in a shallow dish.
4. Sprinkle bread crumbs on wax paper.
5. Dip fish fillets in the yogurt mixture, then coat both sides with bread crumbs.
6. Arrange fish in a single layer on the baking pan and sprinkle with salt, pepper, and paprika.
7. Bake the fish, uncovered for 8 minutes or until coating is light brown.
8. Fish is done when it is flaky.

NUTRITIONAL INFORMATION *(per serving)*:
Calories, 250; carbohydrate, 20 g; protein, 26 g;
fat, 6 g; saturated fat, 1 g; cholesterol, 55 mg; fiber, 1 g;
sodium, 690 mg.

Index